Mapping the Social Consequences of Alcohol Consumption

Mapping the Social Consequences of Alcohol Consumption

Edited by

Harald Klingemann
*Institute for Social Planning and Social Management,
University of Applied Sciences, Bern, Switzerland*

and

Gerhard Gmel
*Swiss Institute for the Prevention of
Alcohol and Other Drug Problems
Lausanne, Switzerland*

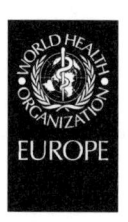

Published on behalf of the World Health Organization Regional Office for Europe
by Kluwer Academic Publishers, Dordrecht, The Netherlands

KLUWER ACADEMIC PUBLISHERS
DORDRECHT / BOSTON / LONDON

Library of Congress Cataloging-in-Publication Data is available.

ISBN 0-7923-6740-5

Published on behalf of the World Health Organization Regional Office for Europe
by Kluwer Academic Publishers,
PO Box 17, 3300 AA Dordrecht, The Netherlands.

Sold and distributed in North, Central and South America
by Kluwer Academic Publishers,101 Philip Drive
Norwell, MA 02018, USA

In all other countries, sold and distributed
by Kluwer Academic Publishers, Distribution Center,
PO Box 322, 3300 AH Dordrecht, The Netherlands

The views expressed in this publication are those of the author(s)/contributors and do not
necessarily represent the decisions or the stated policy of the World Health Organization.

Printed on acid-free paper

All Rights Reserved
© 2001 World Health Organization
No part of this publication may be reproduced or
utilized in any form or by any means, electronic, mechanical,
including photocopying, recording or by any information storage and
retrieval system, without written permission from the copyright owner.

Printed and bound in Great Britain by Antony Rowe Ltd.

Contents

	List of contributors	ix
	Introduction: Social consequences of alcohol – the forgotten dimension? *H. Klingemann and G. Gmel*	1
1.	Concepts, dimensions and measures of alcohol-related social consequences – A basic framework for alcohol-related benefits and harm *J. Rehm*	11
	Measurement issues	15
	References	18
2.	What is meant by 'alcohol-related' consequences? *K. Pernanen*	21
	Alcohol-relatedness: coincidence, common etiology and causality	21
	Social-science and natural-science processes and consequences	22
	Establishing a causal relationship	24
	An alcohol-free society	25
	Determining social consequences	27
	Multiple causal determination	28
	References	31
3.	Alcohol consumption and social harm: quantitative research methodology *G. Gmel and E. Gutjahr*	33
	Assessment of outcome	34
	Assessment of exposure	40
	Covariates: confounding and control variables	41
	Study design	42

	Some less-known designs for investigation of alcohol-related social harm	44
	Conclusions	47
	References	48
4.	**Consequences of drinking to friends and the close social environment** *K. Pernanen*	53
	Friends, social environment	53
	Concluding remarks	62
	References	63
5.	**The impact of alcohol consumption on work and education** *J. Rehm and I. Rossow*	67
	Work	67
	Alcohol and absenteeism	68
	Alcohol-related work problems other than absenteeism	70
	Interaction of alcohol consumption with other factors	70
	Drinking patterns associated with workplace problems	71
	Education	71
	References	74
6.	**Problem drinking and relatives** *E. Maffli*	79
	Introduction	79
	Consequences for children	80
	Consequences for the spouse/partner	84
	Conclusion	86
	References	88
7.	**Accidents, suicide and violence** *I. Rossow, K. Pernanen and J. Rehm*	93
	Introduction	93
	Alcohol and external trauma	94
	Alcohol and accidents	95
	Suicide and parasuicide	98
	Alcohol and violence	100
	Disability and mortality	104
	Summary and implications	105
	References	107

Contents

8. Public order and safety
   H. Klingemann — 113

   The role of alcohol in crime: police and the criminal
   justice system as guardians of 'the public order' — 114
   Compulsory treatment and 'danger to the public':
   treatment and criminal justice cooperating in the
   interests of the public order — 115
   The impact of alcohol consumption on the physical
   and social environment, and communal/municipal
   authorities as representatives of the public order — 117
   Alcohol consumption as part of deviant life-styles?
   Skid rows and the homeless: welfare agencies, social work
   and neighbourhoods with vested interests in public order — 119
   Drinking and occupational careers: conflicts at the
   work-site and discrimination in the labour market — 120
   Public order and cultural aspects: social climate and
   level of tolerance — 121
   Symbolic public display and potential offence to onlookers
   of alcohol as a commodity: moral crusaders defending the
   public order or controlling the poor? — 124
   Drinking and alcohol in youth subcultures: youth and
   alcohol in conflict with the dominant culture (controlling youth) — 125
   Hooliganism – 'episodic' antisocial, delinquent behaviour:
   social workers, politicians and the public as guardians of
   'the public order' — 126
   Concluding remarks: implications for policy makers — 127
   References — 129

9. The social costs of alcohol consumption
   E. Gutjahr and G. Gmel — 133

   What constitutes social costs and how they are estimated — 133
   Recent European and non-European cost estimates — 135
   Policy implications — 140
   References — 142

10. Harm minimization
    M. Plant — 145

    Introduction: What is 'harm minimization'? — 145
    Education — 147
    Community action — 148
    Safer drinking places — 151
    Labelling to warn and inform — 152

Treatment	154
Sustainability	154
Structural control policies	155
Conclusion	156
References	157

11. Community initiatives as strategies for implementation of the European Alcohol Action Plan
    M. Holmila 161

Introduction	161
Examples of reported European projects	164
The Lahti project	164
The Florence Community Alcohol Research project	165
The Kirseberg project	165
The Malczyce Community Action project in Poland	165
The Stad project in Stockholm, Sweden	165
Lessons learned	166
References	168

Contributors

Gmel, Gerhard
Swiss Institute for the Prevention of Alcohol and Other Drug Problems, Lausanne, Switzerland

Gutjahr, Elisabeth
Swiss Institute for the Prevention of Alcohol and Other Drug Problems, Lausanne, Switzerland

Holmila, Marja
Social Research Unit for Alcohol Studies, STAKES, Helsinki, Finland

Klingemann, Harald
Institute for Social Planning and Social Management, University of Applied Sciences, Bern, Switzerland

Maffli, Etienne
Swiss Institute for the Prevention of Alcohol and Other Drug Problems, Lausanne, Switzerland

Pernanen, Kai
National Institute for Alcohol and Drug Research, Oslo, Norway

Plant, Martin
Alcohol and Health Research Centre, City Hospital, Edinburgh, Scotland, United Kingdom

Rehm, Jürgen
Addiction Research Institute, Zürich, Switzerland

Rossow, Ingeborg
National Institute for Alcohol and Drug Research, Oslo, Norway

Introduction:
Social consequences of alcohol – the forgotten dimension?

H. Klingemann and G. Gmel

Health consequences of long-term drinking along with issues of drinking and driving have dominated public discussion on alcohol-related problems. Such social consequences as non-traffic injuries, spouse/family problems, stranger violence, and suicide or attempted suicide have received much less public or research attention. Recent instances of this selective perspective are the report prepared for the Australian Commonwealth Department of Health and Aged Care [1] and the 10th Special Report to the United States Congress on 'Alcohol and Health' [2]. Though the emphasis of the latter report is largely on aspects of neuroscience and biology, including genetics, and on medical consequences, it includes sections on 'Alcohol and Violence', 'Psychosocial Factors' and 'Alcohol-Impaired Driving', in recognition of the relevance of non-medical consequences of alcohol consumption. This may be indicative of a growing interest in a broader concept of alcohol-related consequences, including harm-reduction as a concern of drug/alcohol policy and research [3]. An example of the increasing recognition of alcohol as an agent of social problems is the release by the British Home Office in August 2000 of an action plan entitled *Tackling alcohol related crime, disorder and nuisance* [4]. The scientific community also has been devoting increased attention to the relationship between patterns of consumption and social consequences. Two combined factors are associated with harmful social consequences of drinking: the volume of alcohol consumed, and the frequency of heavy-drinking events. Conferences held in 1995 in Toronto (International Conference on Social and Health Effects of Drinking Patterns) and a follow-up meeting in 1998 in Perth, Australia, have shed more light on these hitherto unexplored issues and highlighted the need to collect more data and improve methods of assessing alcohol-related social outcomes (see a selection of articles

Harald Klingemann and Gerhard Gmel (eds.), Mapping the Social Consequences of Alcohol Consumption, 1–9.
© *2001 Kluwer Academic Publishers. Printed in Great Britain.*

and summaries in Addiction 11, 1996, the thematic issue of Contemporary Drug Problems 3, 1996, and [5, 6]). This leads us to the focus of this book.

Clearly, alcohol has many consequences, harmful as well as beneficial, that can be characterized as 'social' and not medical, or at least only indirectly health-related. This is reflected in the Second European Alcohol Action Plan 2000–2005 of the Regional Office for Europe of the World Health Organization (WHO) [7], designed to prevent or reduce the harm caused by alcohol to the health and well-being of individuals, families and communities.

The present volume is the product of a first attempt to provide a comprehensive overview of the social consequences of alcohol consumption for individuals, groups, organizations and society. It is the outcome of a two-year collaborative project under the leadership of the WHO collaborating centre for substance abuse, research, prevention and documentation (The Swiss Institute for the Prevention of Alcohol and Drug Problems) with the participation of alcohol researchers from Finland, Germany, Norway, Scotland and Switzerland. Its scope, however, is not limited to a regional perspective.

A working meeting of the expert group concerned first took place on the occasion of the annual meeting of the Kettil Bruun Society for Social and Epidemiological Research on Alcohol, in Montreal, Canada in 1999, and a closing workshop was held at Les Diablerets, Switzerland in 2000. At these meetings the group discussed the joint framework and developed a working definition of 'social consequences of alcohol consumption'.

At this point a disclaimer is necessary: The project has been concerned specifically with the descriptive epidemiology of social harm attributable to alcohol consumption. Because of the extensive coverage that this demanded, only two chapters could be devoted to strategies for reducing social harm from alcohol consumption: those on community programmes and harm-reduction measures. Especially in relation to policy, therefore, the book should be seen as complementary to other projects already carried out or under way. Most prominent of these is an updating of the project 'Alcohol Policy and the Public Good', co-sponsored by the WHO Regional Office for Europe, on alcohol problems, including, for the first time, social consequences. A publication from that project is expected in 2001 or 2002 (Oxford University Press). Already appearing this autumn as a special issue of *Addiction* will be the results of the 'Supply Side Initiative', also sponsored by the Regional Office, covering, among other subjects, those of 'alcohol policy and public health' and 'the role of commercial interests in alcohol policies', both of which have implications, positive and negative, for 'social consequences'. Two other activities are relevant in this context: the topical comparative study on alcohol consumption and alcohol problems among women in European countries [8]; ECAS (European Comparative Alcohol Study), which addresses major elements of alcohol policy in the European Union [9, 10]; and efforts to refine measurements (e.g. the Conference in 2000 on 'Measuring Drinking Patterns, Alcohol Problems, and their Connection', at Skarpö, Sweden).

This short and by no means exhaustive overview of projects shows the difficulty of singling out a particular dimension of the complexity of the impact of alcohol consumption on society. The research programme, publication initiatives and task-force efforts in relation to alcohol launched by the Regional Office for Europe have to be seen together, therefore.

Many people claim some understanding of what is meant by 'social consequences' of alcohol consumption. Yet, the establishment of a practical working definition to guide the compilation of the various thematic chapters proved a challenge, taken up in Chapter 1. A negative definition would simply consider all consequences that are not directly medical in nature (e.g. liver cirrhosis from alcohol consumption is *not* a social consequence) and that involve other persons besides the drinker. The working definition finally adopted after long discussion, for purposes of this project, was the following, which takes account of attributional processes and encompasses both negative and positive consequences:

> 'Social consequences of alcohol are changes, subjectively or objectively attributed or attributable to alcohol, occurring in individual social behaviour or in social interaction or in the social environment.'

A second challenge was to arrive at a clearer conception of what is meant by alcohol relatedness – in other words, the idea of causality – in the analysis of social harm. Chapter 2 makes clear that the terms <related to> <associated with> and <linked to>, when used in connection with alcohol consumption and some subsequent social behaviour or action, are sometimes interpreted as implying causality. They mean no more, however, than that when alcohol is present in an event the particular social behaviour or action also tends to occur. It is far from a statement of cause and effect. Even where alcohol appears to be a direct cause of, for instance, a traffic accident, there may be other contributory causes and the net effect of alcohol is difficult to determine. This problem, however, has little to do with the specificities of the 'variable alcohol'; it is connected, rather, with the complexity of accidents. Even if everything has been done, as in the case of a crash of a passenger airplane, the result is often that the 'cause' cannot be determined: there are too many variables. At the same time, alcohol as a chemical substance has predictable properties, which are evident in chemical reactions. Also, it has characteristic effects on the metabolic functions of the human organism. The psychomotor effects of alcohol, on driving skills, for instance, also have consequences for behaviour. They are easy to predict and it is relatively easy to establish when they are caused by alcohol, as police do regularly in roadside checks.

Some of the immediate effects of alcohol on biochemical, metabolic, psychomotor and cognitive processes are responsible for many of its social consequences but, again, they do not suffice for predicting and explaining these consequences in full.

While Chapter 2 warns the reader against applying the label 'alcohol-related' prematurely, Chapter 3 outlines the basic designs and pitfalls to be kept in mind by policy-makers, treatment providers and others concerned with alcohol-related consequences in practice when they declare their decisions and programmes to be 'evidence-based'. After the first, conceptual, part of the book the second part introduces various thematic areas.

ALCOHOL AND THE SOCIAL FABRIC OF GROUPS

Chapter 4 highlights the part that friends play in the social environment in which young people learn how to drink and how to behave after drinking. The influence is mutual: young people are selected to be friends because of their drinking habits and their attitudes towards alcohol; and young people, as well as adults, select their friends in accordance with their own drinking preferences. These processes lead to a certain compatibility with regard to alcohol in networks of friends. When alcohol determines much of the style and content of a person's life, it also becomes a major determinant of friendship networks.

Quality of friendships and the effects of alcohol on friendships should not be judged entirely according to middle-class values. Alcohol-dependent individuals, including those 'on Skid Row', can form intense and supportive friendships. Alcohol induces considerable emotional instability, however, through its effects on the central nervous system and this is reflected in the interaction within such friendship groups. Initiation into certain groups, such as military units or college fraternities, sometimes includes drinking of very large amounts of alcohol, so-called binge drinking. Such drinking carries a high risk of accidental injury, violence and acute alcohol poisoning. It also has implications for the development of problem drinking patterns later in life. Although it is generally believed that alcohol is considered a mitigating factor regarding the attachment of blame or responsibility for the high-risk activities and socially disruptive behaviour associated with such drinking, recent surveys show that the general public does not regard drunkenness as a valid excuse for such behaviour.

Chapter 5 discusses the impact of alcohol consumption on productivity and work career, demonstrated in many studies. Although alcohol consumption does not seem to account for a large proportion of the total production losses from work absenteeism, it is well established that alcohol dependents and heavy drinkers have more sick-leave days than other employees and thus cost their employers considerable amounts (e.g. in Great Britain an estimated £779 million annually). Also, according to some studies, most workers who report sick leave from drinking belong to the large group of more or less moderate drinkers. This kind of alcohol-related absenteeism is probably short-term sick leave due to hangovers from occasional episodes of heavy drinking. Many studies have shown an association between unemployment and heavy drinking.

Alcohol consumption affects education in two ways. One is that parental heavy drinking increases the risk of poor performance of children at school, and of truancy and drop-out. In some cases a mother's heavy drinking during pregnancy leads to attention deficits and behavioural problems in the child. Also, parental heavy drinking (or alcohol abuse) seems to affect parenting skills and, thereby again, the child's school performance. The other is the effect of heavy drinking episodes on the school performance of students and on their educational careers. Some studies have shown that school drop-out is more common among heavy-drinking students than among others.

The relationship between alcohol and domestic violence is linked to spousal/partner and family structures. Chapter 6 makes clear that the prevalence of the problem is often underestimated, for a number of reasons. Legal and cultural limits, for instance, bar access to the private or domestic sphere, even though the physical and psychological well-being of women is at stake, and victims hesitate to report this covert violence.

Although in the current state of knowledge it is difficult to determine the amount of the suffering and harm undergone by the immediate family of the heavy drinker, it is likely to be considerable and at least as great – albeit different in nature – as that of the drinkers themselves. Children are the most severely affected, since they can do little to protect themselves from the direct or indirect consequences of parental drinking. In Western countries, at least one child in 3000 is born with fetal alcohol syndrome, and there is as well a tenfold higher incidence of related disorders linked to direct exposure to alcohol during gestation. Obviously, therefore, parental drinking can seriously harm a child's development, although its modes of action have been only partially elucidated. They involve abuse, neglect, isolation and insecurity, or inconsistent parental behaviour and demands, which are much more common in the families of alcohol abusers than in others. Partners of alcohol-abusers are also at serious risk of violence.

SAFETY, PUBLIC ORDER AND SOCIAL CONTROL OF ALCOHOL-RELATED BEHAVIOUR

There is a great deal of scientific evidence, from numerous research reports, that drinking has a significant impact on accidents, suicide and violence, as Chapter 7 clearly shows. These studies have employed different methods and data from many countries and cultures, and the findings point consistently in the same direction. Drinking to intoxication increases the likelihood of injury from accidents and violence, and of suicide or attempted suicide. From a preventive perspective, it is interesting to note that significant reductions in injuries from accidents and violence, and in suicide, have also been observed when alcohol consumption in a population has decreased, whether as a result of particular policy measures or for other reasons.

In Western societies, since the time of the temperance movement, alcohol has been considered a major cause of deviant behaviour, ranging from disorderly, socially disruptive conduct to serious threats to order and crime. The above-mentioned report of the British Home Office illustrates these issues impressively:

> Alcohol misuse contributes significantly to crime levels, through alcohol specific offences ... against the licensing laws ... or offences committed under the influence of alcohol: it has been estimated that 40% of violent crime, 78% of assaults and 88% of criminal damage cases are committed while the offender is under the influence of alcohol. Alcohol is often consumed by offenders and victims prior to the offence being committed, and it is inextricably linked to disorder around licensed premises [4].

These issues are comprehensively discussed in Chapter 8, which emphasizes at the same time that alcohol control measures to increase public safety and order should be based on evidence rather than morality. Policy measures designed to control 'difficult' or disadvantaged groups (e.g. youth subcultures, the poor and the homeless) by reducing broad socio-political issues to an alcohol-only issue are counterproductive to an efficient alcohol policy with high credibility in the long run. Civil rights have to be respected, especially when implementing so-called 'zero tolerance policies'. Punitive or control measures must not add to cultural or social stigma or have the effect of exposing drinkers to environments that conduce to even more serious social disorder.

In the light of all these perspectives on social problems, Chapter 9 undertakes the difficult task of attaching an economic cost to the social consequences of alcohol consumption.

Alcohol consumption, especially abusive consumption, can entail substantial direct (e.g. welfare expenditures) and indirect (e.g. unemployment) costs to society. Compared with other drugs, such as tobacco or illicit drugs, alcohol is clearly more expensive in terms of resources expended on dealing with the adverse consequences of abusive drinking.

SELECTED STRATEGIES FOR ACTION

Harm reduction as a policy framework – with respect to illicit drugs in particular – has been subject to highly politicized debate and controversy. 'Harm minimization' is limited to the reduction of adverse effects of alcohol. As, for instance, the four-pronged Swiss drug policy, based on repression, treatment,

> The social costs of alcohol consumption amount to between 1% and 3% of Gross Domestic Product.
>
> Thus, for the European Union in 1998, the social costs of alcohol consumption can be estimated at between US$ 64 939 and US$ 194 817 million at constant prices and exchange rates of 1990. About 20% of the total costs are direct costs, representing the amount actually spent for medical, social and judicial services.
>
> About 10% of the total costs are spent on material damage.

harm reduction and prevention, exemplifies, this approach is only one element within complex policy packages. This aspect is stressed also in Chapter 10, which applies a neutral yardstick using the following four questions to assess harm-minimization policies:

- Have those policies worked?
- Are they transferable to other contexts?
- Are they politically and socially acceptable?
- Can they be sustained?

Moreover, the author interprets the concept of harm reduction broadly, in a sense that may be considered debatable.

The companion chapter (Chapter 11), on community action, provides a direct link with the European Alcohol Action Plan, which recognizes the contribution that community programmes and local action can make in supporting healthier lifestyles as well as in securing public and political support for modifying the sale and consumption of alcohol. The author presents – on the basis of international cooperation among community research projects – a broad overview of lessons learned from initiatives and interventions in different countries and cultures.

Available evidence suggests that health promotion may be of value in increasing knowledge about, or changing attitudes towards, alcohol. Moreover, community action has created coalitions of concerned people and reduced crime and disorder, as well as injuries, related to alcohol consumption. It also enhances the quality of life and strengthens services that support problem drinkers and their families.

A core message – regardless of cultural context – is that, despite the enthusiasm, energy and good intentions of those who work in and support prevention, if prevention does not become a part of the routine and regular institutional arrangements of a community, the long-term value of their efforts is often lost. Thus, even if community programmes that initiate preventive action in a community are not sustained, one of their aims should be to bring about policy and structural changes that ensure the institutionalization of measures that promote the health and well-being of the community.

This publication, it is hoped, will serve as a useful source-book for interested policy-makers, specialists in prevention, treatment providers and lay people. At the same time it outlines a research agenda for the future and points to the necessity of more, in-depth, research into the social consequences of alcohol consumption.

Special thanks go to the research centres that made possible the participation of their staff members who contributed to this project; the Kettil Bruun Society for Social and Epidemiological Research on Alcohol, which enabled the working group to meet in Montreal in 1999; and the Swiss Institute for the Prevention of Alcohol and other Drug Problems (SIPA), which organized the 2000 concluding meeting and co-sponsored the project financially. Particular mention should be made of Dr James Gallagher for his assiduous attention to the linguistic quality of this work, and of Ms Elisabeth Grisel and Ms Lucienne Boujon at SIPA, who ensured excellent secretarial back-up. The interest and cooperation of Dr Olaf J. Blaauw, Medical Publishing Editor, Kluwer Academic Publishers, Dordrecht, the Netherlands, and of the Publications Programme of the WHO Regional Office for Europe, Copenhagen, have been highly appreciated throughout this undertaking.

REFERENCES

1. Single, E. et al. (1999) *Evidence regarding the level of alcohol consumption considered to be low-risk for men and women.* Australian Commonwealth Department of Health and Aged Care, Canberra (Final Report).
2. United States Department of Health and Human Services. (2000) *10th Special Report to the US Congress on Alcohol and Health from the Secretary of Health and Human Services.* US Department of Health and Human Services, Public Health Services, National Institutes of Health, National Institute on Alcohol Abuse and Alcoholism, Washington, (NIH Publications, No. 00-1583.2000).
3. Stockwell, T. et al. (1997) Sharpening the focus of alcohol policy from aggregate consumption to harm and risk reduction. *Addiction Research* 5(1), 1–9.
4. Home Office. (2000) Tackling alcohol related crime, disorder and nuisance. *Action Plan*: http://www.homeoffice.gov.uk/pcrg/aap0700.htm
5. Rehm, J. and Gmel, G. (1999) Patterns of alcohol consumption and social consequences. Results from an 8-year follow-up study in Switzerland. *Addiction* 94(6), 899–912.
6. Rehm, J. and Gmel, G. (2000) Gaps and needs in international alcohol epidemiology. *Journal of Substance Use* 5, 6–13.
7. *Second European Alcohol Action Plan 2000–2005.* Copenhagen: World Health Organization Regional Office for Europe, 2000 (document EUR/LVNG 01 05 01).

8. Bloomfield, K. *et al.* (1999) *Alcohol Consumption and Alcohol Problems among Women in European Countries.* Institute for Medical Informatics, Biostatistics and Epidemiology, Free University of Berlin, Berlin, (Project Final Report).
9. Norström, T. (1999) European comparative alcohol study – ECAS. Project presentation. *Nordic Studies on Alcohol and Drugs* **16**, 5–6.
10. Holder, H. *et al.* (1998) *European Integration and Nordic Alcohol Policies – Changes in Alcohol Controls and Consequences in Finland, Norway and Sweden, 1980–1997.* Brookfield, Ashgate.

Chapter one

Concepts, dimensions and measures of alcohol-related social consequences – A basic framework for alcohol-related benefits and harm

J. Rehm

As outlined in Table 1, I am suggesting a conceptual framework of categories of consequences related to the use of alcohol, which consists of two basic dimensions [1–3, 13, for similar earlier efforts, although restricted to harm].

First, we suggest distinguishing between different categories of consequences – acute and long-term (in the literature often referred to as chronic consequences). Clearly, the consequences to the user and the user's environment of a single experience with any drug are different from those of a pattern of repeated use over time – a pattern that may, in the extreme, last almost a life-time.

Second, we are suggesting four major functional areas in which consequences may follow from the use of alcohol (columns of Table 1):

- The individual's physiological health;
- The individual's psycho-physiological and mental health;

Harald Klingemann and Gerhard Gmel (eds.), Mapping the Social Consequences of Alcohol Consumption, 11–19.
© *2001 Kluwer Academic Publishers. Printed in Great Britain.*

Table 1 Conceptual scheme of categories of harm and benefits from alcohol for single-occasion and long-term use

	Physiological health	Psycho-physiological and mental	Immediate personal and social environment (behavioural aspect)	Wider social and cultural level (determined by societal reaction)
Harm				
Single-occasion use (= acute consequences)	Overdose	Changed consciousness and control (hangover/suicide); injury to drinker and others	Severe family and workplace disruption, injury to others, violence	Formal (legal ≥ criminalization) and informal sanctions
Long-term use (= chronic consequences)	Increase of mortality (liver cirrhosis); morbidity, disability for certain patterns of use	Dependence, depression	Disruption of social and economic relations	Stigmatization; coercion to change; treatment; criminalization of alcohol-related behaviour; associated costs
Benefits				
Single-occasion use (= acute consequences)	Relaxation	Feeling less stress and subjectively well	Improving social events	Cultural identification and integration, benefits from taxation
Long-term use (= chronic consequences)	Mortality, morbidity and disability reduction if used regularly and moderately	General subjective well-being, cognitive functioning	Group cohesion	

(Harm part adapted from Rehm and Fischer [2], with examples in each table cell)

- The immediate personal and social environment and the drinker's social and economic relations, including especially the environment of family, friends and peers, as well as work-places and public spaces;
- The larger societal level and its mostly institutionalized societal reactions to alcohol use and related harm and benefits.

In addition to this, in the social sciences, consequences of alcohol are discussed, where alcohol is only socially constructed to be part of a social process or event even though it may not play such a role in reality.

At the individual level, alcohol produces negative as well as positive physiological and psycho-physiological or mental effects (for overviews [4–6]). Most of these would fall within categories of the International Classification of Diseases (ICD), either relating different patterns of consumption to defined mortality and morbidity outcomes by epidemiological studies [7] or by extending the definition of harmful use by analogy to beneficial effects. This definition states that there must be '… clear evidence that the substance use was responsible for (…) physical or psychological harm (…) which may lead to disability or have adverse consequences for interpersonal relationships' [8, p 56; 9, pp. 74–75 for an earlier, more narrow definition]. This definition requires a causal relationship between alcohol and outcomes (see Chapter 2 for further discussion).

In addition to individual-level consequences, we propose two fundamental dimensions in which alcohol use can produce positive and negative consequences, benefits and harm to others as well as to society more generally. These dimensions would cover social consequences in the strict sense. The first comprises the immediate personal and social environment and the drinker's social and economic relations, including especially the environment of family, friends and peers, as well as workplaces and public spaces. The effects of alcohol on this environment are determined mainly by the inherent properties of alcohol, regardless of contingent or reactive circumstances, or by the interaction between these effects and reactions of the immediate environment to drinking. Violence against others and decreased productivity are examples of harm in this category; they are related primarily to the drug's inherent mind-altering and other qualities (see, for example, the discussion on alcohol and violence [10]).

The second dimension consists of the larger societal level and its mostly institutionalized societal reactions to alcohol use and related harms and benefits.

These reactions to alcohol use – designed mostly to prevent and control harm from behaviour related to alcohol use (viz., criminal and regulatory laws) – account for part of the negative consequences and costs that arise in relation to alcohol use. At the same time, alcohol brings social benefits such as tax revenue from alcoholic beverages or employment provided by the alcohol industry, and this has to be taken into account in any discussion of social consequences of alcohol consumption.

This category of 'reacting' variables at the societal level also produces significant harm to the alcohol user (and to society), through, for example, stigmatization or social exclusion (criminalization) as a reaction to individual drinking, or positive processes of social integration or identification facilitated by drinking. These reactions, and the harm, costs or benefits attributable to them, are not primarily inherent to alcohol or its use – they are ideological, social and cultural. Examples of harm and costs in this respect include the criminalization of alcohol use in restricted locations, under a certain age, or in correlation with violence or driving; the stigma often attached to drinkers; and various forms of social control and pressure from (often medical) treatment systems to change alcohol-related behaviour.

It may be argued that the principal categories of alcohol-related harm and benefits suggested are not necessarily closely linked – that outcomes related to one category can occur without outcomes related to another. In practice, however, outcomes in these basic conceptual categories often relate to one another. Thus, the patho-physiological and mental effects of drinking on individuals are largely the cause of loss of productivity as a form of social harm from alcohol use. The harms and benefits at the 'societal level' are often a reaction to those in the category of social and individual harm and benefits that are inherent to alcohol.

The definition of social consequences as discussed so far, however, has included only the parts of social harm which could be defined in a positivist way. Other consequences of drinking are social constructions that are part of a social process or events in which alcohol is socially constructed to be part of a social process or event. If this category of social harm is included as well, we end up with the following definition of social consequences, to be applied in this book:

'Social consequences of alcohol are changes, subjectively or objectively attributed or attributable to alcohol, occurring in individual social behaviour or in social interaction or in the social environment.'

Changes can be positively, negatively or neutrally evaluated by the individual and the interaction partners of the individual. Some of these changes may be expressed in economic costs.

Social behaviour is behaviour oriented to others with social meaning attributed, in the sense of M. Weber [11].

Interaction refers to cases in which:

- the individual is directly implicated, and concerned by the social response (partner leaving, dismissal from work, relatives trying to educate drinking pregnant women).

- the changes in interaction are on the aggregate/system level (discrimination and labelling of alcoholics or changing economic conditions).

Circumstances refer to the environment without necessarily implying change due to interaction.

Subjective attribution refers to cases in which subjects see behavioural change as related to alcohol (including self-handicapping), regardless of whether the role of alcohol can be confirmed by scientific rules (which would refer to **objectively attributable**).

Perhaps the best way to further illustrate this definition is by examples of what is included or excluded. The above definition does not cover cirrhosis of the liver as a long-term biological consequence of alcohol consumption (see also Table 1, and the attached descriptions). Social consequences, however, do include changes in social behaviour triggered by liver cirrhosis (such as discontinued attendance at parties because one has stopped drinking), changes in interaction (such as different patterns of interaction with a partner), and changes in circumstances (such as a disability pension). This example is intended to illustrate that the consequences mainly excluded by the definition are the purely biological.

MEASUREMENT ISSUES

In aiming at a comprehensive audit of alcohol-related outcomes, especially social benefits and harm, the critical questions are:

- For what outcomes do we have solid evidence about the relation between alcohol and outcome?

- For what outcomes of alcohol-related benefits and harms do solid data indicators exist?

An inspection of the categories listed in Table 1 reveals that the most solid data indicators are those that refer to the physiological and mental/psychophysiological consequences of alcohol use, especially for mortality [12].[1] The data on alcohol-related mortality are, in general, sophisticated and mostly comparable, at least in industrialized countries.

---

[1] Mortality statistics also contribute to part of the second column (mortality from accidents and injuries; ICD 9 E-codes). In most industrialized countries the alcohol-related morbidity and mortality from accidents and injuries outweigh morbidity and mortality from more physiologically related categories like cirrhosis or cancers.

16 Concepts, dimensions and measures of alcohol-related social consequences

The indicators, however, do not usually measure directly the fraction of the mortality attributable to alcohol, which varies widely between societies.[2] Exceptions here are disease categories that are, by definition, 100% attributable to alcohol, such as alcohol dependence or alcohol psychosis. The trend in constructing international classification systems for diseases, however, seems to go in the direction of defining diseases on the basis of signs and symptoms, irrespective of etiology (e.g. the DSM IV system).

The indicators for alcohol-related morbidity are also fairly comprehensive in industrialized countries (see the various cost studies: for an overview [13]).

People who suffer from health consequences of alcohol use tend normally to make use of comprehensive health and medical services, which function as acceptable sources of records on such data.

There are some indicators of the negative effects from changed mental states due to alcohol use on a single occasion, in particular because of the legal and accounting systems that track accidents after drinking-driving or other accidents, or the tracking of law-breaking in criminal justice systems. Again, usually only the criminal incidents are recorded, irrespective of cause or reason (specific statistics on alcohol-related road accidents are the most notable exception in most industrialized countries). Little is known about the negative contingencies of potential 'dependence' of long-term drinkers.

Especially in this area, there are also vast cultural differences in the definition of events procedures [Reference 14, and the subsequent commentary series].

As regards medical consequences, most data deficiencies relate to disability [15], regrettably a condition relatively more linked to alcohol than mortality or morbidity [16]. Both solid research to quantify the effect of alcohol [17] and data on prevalence or incidence of disability [18] are needed.

The available data indicators on consequences to the direct social and personal environment from short-term as well as long-term use of alcohol are sparse and inconsistent. Drinking, whether in the short or the long term, can have distressing consequences for friends and for family and other social relations [19]. Also, heavy use of alcohol can disrupt people's lifestyles as well as their personal relationships, but there are no standard measures or data that would permit those consequences to be quantified in a comparable manner, nor are there sources of standardized and reliable data on the quantification of alcohol-related benefits to the immediate environment. Finally, the relatively sparse research into the relationship between alcohol and consequences in the drinker's direct social environment often employs faulty methods, such as the use of a single survey question to ask about both cause and consequence (see Chapter 3; also [15], for a more detailed discussion).

---

[2] Attributable fractions for alcohol for different causes of mortality vary most drastically for causes of death heavily influenced by the social context, such as suicide or road accidents, but there is also variation in such causes as liver cirrhosis: in some parts of the world non-alcoholic liver cirrhosis rates are quite substantial whereas in others this category is almost extinct.

The quantification of social costs and monetary benefits to society has been proposed and used as the best approach to determining social consequences of alcohol use [20–22; see also Chapter 10]. Many consequences can be accounted for in some form of material 'cost', since they are established by a formalized societal intervention entailing a defined amount of expenses or compensation to be paid out of the public purse [23, for an overview].[3] These negative, societally determined consequences, are, by definition, social in nature, as a form of social reaction that predominantly reflects an institutionalized system of values, actors or mechanisms designed to control behaviour. It is not inherently criminal to make excessive noise after drinking or to drink in a public park, but a country's legal system criminalizes such behaviour. A selected mode of social control makes the drinker a criminal, and thus harms the individual as well as the societal context (see Chapter 8).

First, however, not all social benefits and harms are so easily quantifiable in monetary terms as criminalized behaviour (e.g. pain, pleasure); and second, all cost studies are only as good as the underlying epidemiological and other sources of data. Any cost study will thus have to cope with the questions and problems outlined above.

Despite their obvious conceptual significance, the conventional ways of accounting for 'harm' and 'benefit' from alcohol use have mostly not yet operationalized the various forms of 'harm' and 'benefit' that occur at the personal/social/economic level or that are due to societal reactions. Ways have yet to be found to incorporate the disruption of families or the social relations of drinkers into the calculation; and a conceptually solid framework grounded in societal responses to alcohol use has yet to be devised for accounting for harm or benefit. The largely institutionalized responses of social control, including legal penalties, control of availability, and treatment measures, as well as such social processes as labelling and the stigmatization of alcohol users, have largely been taken for granted as being inherent, and directly linked, to alcohol use. These responses, it must be recognized, came about as a societal reaction to the consumption of alcohol, mostly gradually, over a long time. Here, conceptually, the social epidemiology of alcohol-related harm stands at the same paradigmatic threshold as criminology some 25 years ago, when labelling or reaction- theory concepts of crime held that the harmful property of crime was not necessarily inherent to some forms of behaviour but, rather, a result of a reaction to such behaviour on the part of society [24, 25]. This becomes crucial if our thinking is to be advanced on how to reduce alcohol-related harm and increase benefit (see Chapter 10). We shall then realize that 'harm reduction' in this sense will mean not only that the alcohol consumer changes behaviour but, equally, that society will modify its reaction to alcohol consumption and alcohol-related behaviour.

---

[3] On a conceptual level harm and costs should be distinguished. However, operational costs are the major and often the only indicator for harm at this level.

REFERENCES

1. Fischer, B. et al. (1997) Charting WHO-goals for licit and illicit drugs for the year 2000: are we 'on track'? *Public Health* **111**, 271–275.
2. Rehm, J. and Fischer, B. (1997) Measuring harm: implications for alcohol epidemiology, in *Alcohol: Minimising the Harm: What Works?* (eds M.A. Plant et al.), Free Association Books, London, pp. 248–261.
3. Room, R. (1985) Alcohol as a cause: empirical links and social definitions, in *Currents in Alcohol Research and the Prevention of Alcohol Problems* (eds J.-P. Von Wartburg et al.), Huber, Berne, pp. 11–19.
4. English, D.R. et al. (1995) *The Quantification of Drug Caused Morbidity and Mortality in Australia*, Commonwealth Department of Human Services and Health, Canberra.
5. Single, E. et al. (1999) *Evidence Regarding the Level of Alcohol Consumption Considered to be Low-Risk for Men and Women*, Australian Commonwealth Department of Health and Aged Care, Canberra1(Final Report).
6. Single, E. et al. (1999) Morbidity and mortality attributable to alcohol, tobacco, and illicit drug use in Canada. *American Journal of Public Health* **89**(3), 385–390.
7. Rothman, K.J. and Greenland, S. (eds) (1998) *Modern Epidemiology*, Lippincott-Raven, Philadelphia, PA.
8. WHO. (1993) *The ICD-10 Classification of Mental and Behavioural Disorders. Diagnostic Criteria for Research*, World Health Organization, Geneva.
9. WHO. (1992) *The ICD-10 Classification of Mental and Behavioural Disorders. Clinical Descriptions and Diagnostic Guidelines*, World Health Organization, Geneva.
10. Graham, K., Leonard, K.E., Room, R. et al. (1998) Current directions in research on understanding and preventing intoxicated aggression. *Addiction* **93**(5), 659–76.
11. Weber, M. (1980) *Wirtschaft und Gesellschaft: Grundriss der verstehenden Soziologie*, J.C.B. Mohr, Tübingen (Paul Siebeck).
12. Murray, C.J.L. and Lopez, A.D. (1996) Quantifying the burden of disease and injury attributable to ten major risk factors, in *Global Burden of Disease: A Comprehensive Assessment of Mortality and Disability from Diseases, Injuries, and Risk Factors in 1990 and Projected to 2020* (eds C.J.L. Murray and A.D. Lopez), Harvard School of Public Health, Cambridge, MA, pp. 295–324.
13. Robson, L. and Single, E. (1995) *Literature Review of Studies on the Economic Costs of Substance Abuse*, Canadian Centre on Substance Abuse, Ottawa.
14. Room, R. et al. (1996) WHO cross-cultural applicability research on diagnosis and assessment of substance use disorders: an overview of methods and selected results. *Addiction* **91**, 199–220 (with commentary series pp. 221–230).
15. Rehm, J. and Gmel, G. (2000) Gaps and needs in international alcohol epidemiology. *Journal of Substance Use* **5**, 6–13.
16. Murray, C. and Lopez, A. (1997) Global mortality, disability, and the contribution of risk factors: global burden of disease study. *Lancet* **349**, 1436–1442.
17. Ashley, M.J. et al. (2000) Health risk and benefits of alcohol consumption: balancing disparate relationships for individual and population health, in *National Institute on Alcohol Abuse and Alcoholism, ed: 10th Special Report to the US Congress on Alcohol and Health*. Rockville, MD, US Department of Health and Human Services, National Institute on Alcohol Abuse and Alcoholism.
18. Goerdt, A. et al. (1996) Non-fatal health outcomes: concepts, instruments and indicators, in *Global Burden of Disease: A Comprehensive Assessment of Mortality and Disability from Diseases, Injuries, and Risk Factors in 1990 and Projected to 2020* (eds C.J.L. Murray and A.D. Lopez), Harvard School of Public Health, Cambridge, MA, pp. 201–246.
19. Pernanen, K. (1991) *Alcohol in Human Violence*. Guilford Press, New York.

20. Collins, D. and Lapsley, H. (1991) *Estimating the Economic Costs of Drug Abuse in Australia*, Commonwealth of Australia, Canberra, (No. 15).
21. Single, E. *et al.* (1988) The economic costs of alcohol, tobacco and illicit drugs in Canada, 1992. *Addiction* **93**(7), 991–1006.
22. Harwood, H.J. *et al.* (1999) Cost estimates for alcohol and drug abuse. *Addiction* **94**(5), 631–635.
23. Xie, X. *et al.* (1996) *The Economic Costs of Alcohol, Tobacco and Illicit Drug Abuse in Ontario: 1992*, Addiction Research Foundation, Toronto (ARF Research Document Series No. 127).
24. Becker, H. (1973) *Outsiders*, Free Press, Glencoe, Ill.
25. Goode, E. (1984) *Deviant Behaviour*, Prentice Hall, Englewood Cliffs.

Chapter two

What is meant by 'alcohol-related' consequences?

K. Pernanen

ALCOHOL-RELATEDNESS: COINCIDENCE, COMMON ETIOLOGY AND CAUSALITY

To say that some condition or incident is *alcohol-related* is to imply (1) that it tends to cluster in time and place with the use of alcohol (being in a statistical sense 'associated' with the use of alcohol); or, more strongly, (2) that alcohol is a risk factor for it; or, even more strongly, (3) that it is caused by alcohol. It is important to distinguish between these meanings and to clarify which type of relationship to alcohol is intended.

Chance association

In some cases an association between alcohol and a social occurrence arises merely by chance. If, for instance, competitive games, such as card or pool games, increase the risk of personal violence and, for traditional or economic reasons, they are held more often in public drinking places than in places where alcohol is not consumed, drinking would then be related by chance to personal violence, although the link between the violence and alcohol need not be causal.[1]

---

[1] Even in such an instance there may be links at some level of causation, such as at the level of cultural meaning, where drinking could have a symbolic affinity with aggression.

Harald Klingemann and Gerhard Gmel (eds.), *Mapping the Social Consequences of Alcohol Consumption*, 21–31.
© 2001 *Kluwer Academic Publishers. Printed in Great Britain.*

Third-factor explanations

In some alcohol-related cases *both* drinking and the related condition or instance of social harm have a common cause, giving rise to a so-called 'spurious relationship'. Such is the case, for instance, if stress or frustration causes people to drink but also gives rise to violent behaviour. Alcohol consumption and violent behaviour would then be seen to be associated, but neither would be a cause of the other. The violence would not be a social consequence of alcohol use, but by the weak use of the term 'alcohol-related' (implying only statistical association) the violent behaviour is called 'alcohol-related'.

Alcohol as a risk factor

When we do not have a sufficiently clear view of the causal mechanisms involved, or if the causal processes are not particularly relevant to our concerns, we speak of alcohol as a risk factor. For example, when there is strong evidence that alcohol consumption leads in *some way* to promiscuous behaviour, and we want to prevent such behaviour in order to stop the spread of sexually transmitted diseases, we tend to speak of alcohol as a risk factor (or, sometimes, as a 'contributory cause'). Speaking of 'risks' indicates that preventive, and not causal or explanatory, concerns are in the foreground.

Causal relationships

Other occurrences have at least a partial causal relationship with alcohol. Some can be said to be consequences of drinking. How to distinguish these from other kinds of relationship is our concern in this chapter. A complication is that what is considered to be a chance relationship and what is a consequence of drinking depends on whether one is prepared to accept that relationships mediated by cultural definitions are 'causal'.

SOCIAL-SCIENCE AND NATURAL-SCIENCE PROCESSES AND CONSEQUENCES

It is useful to distinguish between consequences of alcohol use that are brought about by natural science (mainly biological) processes and those that are caused by the mental and social processes linked to alcohol use. Liver damage from drinking is an example of natural (biological) consequences. It is much easier to predict natural (biological) than social processes and consequences. Some of the natural processes and consequences must be taken into account in order to explain and predict social consequences.

By 'social consequence' of alcohol use we here mean a condition that recurs with some regularity in connection with, or at some point after, the consumption of alcohol.

On the basis of the regularity there must also be good evidence that *some aspect or property* of alcohol has led to that consequence in a sufficient number of cases. Instances of various properties of alcohol could be its pharmacological effects, or the cue value of a bottle containing (presumably) an alcoholic beverage, or the cues linked to being present in a drinking establishment, or the cultural connotations of alcohol (as when it symbolizes rebelliousness or permissiveness). The other chapters of this book will give a good idea of the range of what are considered to be social consequences of alcohol consumption.

Natural-level effects of alcohol have social consequences if they affect the social life of individuals. Liver damage will make demands on health services, and family relationships will be affected. The effects of alcohol on cognitive abilities such as attention, perception and information processing, as well as psychomotor disturbances, will affect social interaction. Addictive properties of alcohol will cause family disruption, work-related problems and ill-health. Some economic aspects of these consequences have been included in calculations of economic costs of alcohol consumption to society [1]. Several important social consequences, the so-called 'intangible' costs, cannot, however, be easily measured in economic terms. They may be characterized as consequences of alcohol consumption for the *quality of life* of individuals.

Alcohol induces some clearly observable psychomotor disturbances: a staggering gait, slurred speech, glazed eyes, a shifty look. They are so indicative of intoxication that police have used them to test whether people suspected of drinking and driving are in fact intoxicated. They also play a part in accidents and trauma related to alcohol use. Psychomotor and cognitive effects are central in bringing about the social consequences of alcohol consumption. In addition to such acute effects, the addictive potential of alcohol, which is based on a mix of natural, mental and social processes of drinking, entails serious social consequences.

Alcohol has also more direct social effects, most obviously patterns of social behaviour and interaction. They are less predictable than psychomotor disturbances. Intoxicated social behaviour may be easy to recognize; its recognition depends very much on concomitant psychomotor cues of the same kind that police use for determining alcohol intoxication and not so much on a specific character or content of social interaction under the influence of alcohol.

Unlike natural-process consequences of drinking, direct social consequences differ between cultures. In many Western societies quarrelsome or overly sentimental behaviour is customary, with perhaps sudden fluctuations. In others – pre-industrial societies in particular – there is wide variation in customary behaviour after drinking [2]. Changes occur over time even in typical drunken behaviour in the same society. There is disagreement, consequently, as to which social consequences are related to the beverage alcohol itself and which to beliefs about alcohol and its symbolic value, its expected effects, and the circumstances in which drinking takes place. Intoxication is most likely to be only one among many factors that determine behaviour after drinking and its social consequences.

Statements on causality differ in strength. The strongest would assert that alcohol is both a sufficient and a necessary cause of an outcome. If alcohol were a necessary condition of liver cirrhosis, the condition would not occur if alcohol was never consumed. If, however, drinking were a sufficient condition, no other factor would need to be taken into account: it would be enough that drinking occurred. Such categorical views are very rare among those who do research into the social consequences of alcohol. The prevailing view is, rather, that other factors besides alcohol are active in determining social consequences linked to alcohol (that is, alcohol is not a sufficient precondition), and that the consequences can come about via some other processes in which alcohol and its effects need not be included (that is, alcohol is not a necessary precondition).

ESTABLISHING A CAUSAL RELATIONSHIP[2]

As with other social consequences, the evidence for a causal relationship with alcohol is especially strong if several fields of inquiry using several different types of methodology point unambiguously to the existence of a relationship. The clearest cases of alcohol-caused conditions are those for which a natural *process* has been found which mediates between alcohol consumption and the particular consequence.

Liver damage is a relatively simple instance of a biological consequence of alcohol consumption. Several types of study point to a causal connection. There is, for instance, epidemiological evidence that populations that consume large amounts of alcohol have a higher than average incidence and prevalence of liver cirrhosis. In addition, there is clinical evidence that heavy drinkers are at high risk of liver damage. Autopsies on deceased alcoholics support this conclusion. Decisive support is provided if the physiological mechanisms by which alcohol or its metabolites affect the particular bodily organ can be specified.[3] The processes by which alcohol produces social effects are more complicated; in establishing causality, several different types of causal influence must be considered.

Minimum alcohol levels

In research on the social consequences of alcohol consumption it is often assumed that *any* amount of alcohol will justify the label 'alcohol-related'. This happens in many surveys when a minimum level of consumption is not

---

[2] The common methodologies used in testing causal hypotheses are not discussed here. They are described in any standard textbook on research methodology. Here the focus is on the long-term research strategies that gradually provide strengthened support for alcohol having a significant causal role in some social and cultural occurrences.

[3] Research on cigarette smoking and lung cancer is a notable example of how findings from different scientific disciplines using various methodologies combined to establish that smoking was indeed a major cause of lung cancer.

specified. In order not to miss a single instance of alcohol association, researchers sometimes even include occurrences in and around public drinking places as alcohol-related even though nothing is known about the alcohol consumption at that time of the people involved. This may be justified on the ground that some social theories of alcohol-relatedness do not require that a single drop of alcohol has been consumed, as is evident from research on alcohol-related expectancies.[4]

The distinction between natural and social consequences is useful for analytical and theoretical purposes. In practice the distinction becomes artificial and blurred. Natural processes affect social occurrences but, conversely, social factors influence the nature and extent of natural processes. Tradition and culture related to the use of alcohol determine, *inter alia*, the availability of alcohol and the average level of alcohol consumption, the nature and frequency of events at which alcohol is used, the alcohol content of the beverages consumed, and beliefs about the effects of alcohol.

AN ALCOHOL-FREE SOCIETY

Probably a good way to understand the wide range of relationships that alcohol consumption has with social experiences or occurrences is to adopt from social economics the concept of an 'alcohol-free society'. In assessing the social costs and benefits of some social item, such as tobacco, drugs or alcohol, it is customary to conceptualize a 'counterfactual scenario' [1].

In assessing the social costs of alcohol a counterfactual situation is used for making comparisons with the actual state of affairs in a society. This situation is defined as a state that would obtain if there were no alcohol in society.

Ideally, comparison of the actual state of a society with the hypothesized counterfactual scenario shows the *net* effect of all positive and negative consequences of alcohol consumption. This logic indicates what social conditions are alcohol-related – that is, they would not have occurred had there been no alcohol consumption in the population. Reference to causality has a tendency to narrow one's focus to the paradigm of natural-science causality. The appeal of the idea of an alcohol-free society for comparison with prevailing conditions is that it does not rule out any types of causal connection and accepts that several types of alcohol-related process underlie social consequences of alcohol use. It is, therefore, a good starting point for raising central questions pertaining to alcohol-relatedness and the social consequences of alcohol use.

---

[4] In alcohol expectancy research, experimental subjects are told that the liquid they are drinking contains alcohol when in fact it does not, and that it is a non-alcoholic beverage when it actually contains alcohol. At least at relatively low consumption levels it is possible to deceive subjects according to these instructions. The results of many experiments show that the belief that one is consuming alcohol has a strong effect on subsequent behaviour.

Consider this scenario: Someone pretends to be drunk, staggers, slurs his speech and mutters to himself in the hope that others will excuse his violent behaviour towards his wife. Would it even be possible in an alcohol-free society to indulge in such behaviour without the risk of being taken in for a psychiatric examination? Can such behaviour be considered a social consequence of alcohol use? Apparently not, if the pharmacological effects of alcohol are considered worthy of consideration in assigning alcohol-relatedness. There is no doubt, however, that in the sphere of cultural beliefs such behaviour has a non-trivial association with alcohol. Cultural beliefs and patterns of behaviour in relation to alcohol have their origins in both acute and long-term effects of drinking. In addition, when alcohol becomes a symbolic and cultural entity it interacts with other general themes in the cultural system.

The closest approximation to an alcohol-free society comes about through sudden restrictions on the availability of alcohol. This occurs, for instance, when strikes in the distribution chain or significant price rises decrease availability. Several of these so-called 'natural' experiments have been short-lived, however, and could not be used to assess longer-term effects of extreme changes in alcohol consumption. Also, the social consequences of more long-lasting restrictions on alcohol sales are difficult to distinguish from those of other, concurrent changes. This is well exemplified by the many confounding experiences that characterized the Prohibition periods in several European countries and the United States.[5]

Important social consequences of alcohol consumption are 'intangible' – that is, they are linked to subjective feelings of wellbeing or discomfort. In monetary values they cannot be so easily measured as the so-called 'real costs'. In an attempt to make them more objectively measurable they have been studied under the concept of quality of life.

Since so little is known about what an alcohol-free society would be like, and in order to arrive at an approximation of what the different social consequences of drinking are, we must be content with trying to piece together the causal studies that have been conducted. This method will be illustrated by the evidence for causal relationships between alcohol consumption and violent behaviour.

---

[5] There are also open questions regarding the historical effects in a society where alcohol disappears after having been consumed over a lengthy period of time. How would a society that has been alcohol-free for one year differ from one that has been free for 10 years? And would the social consequences be taken over by some other substance or some other processes? Were they truly 'alcohol-related' in the sense that they were specific to alcohol?

DETERMINING SOCIAL CONSEQUENCES

It is not easy to determine whether a social occurrence that is associated with alcohol use is a consequence of such use, as can be illustrated by the difficulties of trying to determine whether violence associated with alcohol is indeed caused by alcohol.

Alcohol being a *chemical* compound with well-established *psychological* and *social* effects, the question of causality becomes multidisciplinary. Researchers from several disciplines are engaged in research designed to answer questions about the type of alcohol-relatedness that may be involved in violent behaviour (and, more generally, to determine what social conditions are caused, at least in part, by alcohol consumption).

The contention that a significant proportion of alcohol-associated violence is indeed alcohol-caused is based on many different kinds of research:

- A great many studies in many parts of the world have shown that alcohol is involved in large proportions of violent crime [3, 4] and of cases of injury from violence that attend medical facilities [5];

- Time series analyses carried out predominantly in Scandinavian countries indicate that rates of violent crime rates are in some countries strongly determined by the level of alcohol consumption in the population [6];

- Sudden changes in the availability of alcohol (so-called 'natural experiments') are followed by corresponding changes in the rate of violent crime and in the numbers of people presenting at medical facilities with injuries from violence [7, 8];

- Many psychological experiments show that the level of alcohol in the blood is directly related to the risk of aggressive behaviour [9, 10].

Violent behaviour is probably the best researched area among the possible social consequences of drinking. Still there is no wide agreement regarding the nature of the link. There is some conflicting evidence from:

- psychological experiments, showing that people's expectancies regarding the effects of alcohol on their mood and behaviour can have a stronger effect on behaviour than levels of blood alcohol;

- anthropological accounts which show considerable variability in post-drinking behaviour in different societies and in the same society over time [2, 11];

- time series analyses, showing that European countries differ greatly in the strength of the relationship between per capita alcohol consumption and rates of violent crime [6];

- studies on violence – in particular, domestic violence – showing that alcohol intoxication is used mainly as an excuse for committing planned violent acts.

To resolve such apparent discrepancies it would have to be accepted that there is nothing necessary or sufficient in the causal relationships that bring about alcohol-related violence, and also that alcohol acts at several levels in causing violence.

MULTIPLE CAUSAL DETERMINATION

Numerous types of causal process are at work in creating the sum total of social consequences of alcohol consumption in a society. Some researchers may object to calling all of them 'causal', but their inclusion is in keeping with our wide definition of the concept of causality, derived from the idea of an alcohol-free society. The main types of such causal influence are:

(1) *Pharmacological effects.* This link is exemplified by the psychomotor and cognitive impairment processes discussed earlier. Alcohol causes misperceptions; it amplifies the significance of minor occurrences in the social environment; it forces the drinker to focus on the here-and-now [12]. This increases the risk of conflict and aggression. The causal role of pharmacological effects is also contained in the idea of the pharmacological 'disinhibition' caused by alcohol.

(2) *Expectancy effects.* The most straightforward of the cue values of alcohol and circumstances linked to drinking are brought out in the expectancy effects of alcohol found in balanced placebo experiments. The experimental subjects are deceived into believing that they are consuming alcohol when they are not and vice versa. The placebo design collapses at relatively low levels of blood alcohol because the subject does not perceive the expected physiological experience. Expectancies may still be active even at higher levels, and the 'tone', mood and interactional themes of a drinking event may be already set with the early expectancy effects. There are both cultural and individual variations in the cue value of alcohol: some expectancies are based on personal experiences with alcohol, and others are based on cultural belief systems regarding alcohol and its effects.

(3) *Motivational/instrumental use.* People sometimes use alcohol to enable them, through its pharmacological effects, to violate everyday social norms. The same type of rule-breaking behaviour can be justified by general expectancies, such as cultural 'time out' definitions of drinking events that take place in some cultures and subcultures. The 'excuse function' of alcohol consumption is part of this cultural configuration.

(4) *Alcohol as part of a cultural-semiotic system.* The symbolism associated with such concepts as mother, father, sex, food and many other 'cultural objects' is central to the understanding of how people reason and behave. In most cultures this symbolism encompasses a wide range of beliefs and provides signals for culturally determined scripts for behaviour. The psychoactive properties of alcohol make it a suitable object for deeper cultural meanings, sometimes assigning supernatural status to the drink and linkage to the divine (cf. being possessed by 'spirits'). Such cultural beliefs define the experience of intoxication to the intoxicated person, and in this way determine the person's thought content and behaviour. To some, alcohol is a symbol of sin and debauchery; to others it stands for revelry and 'time-out'. For youth it is often a symbol of rebellion, freedom and adulthood.

In common with many other human activities and experiences in the social environment, alcohol, drinking, and drunkenness determine behaviour through several types of social process. Even one and the same instance of a social consequence, such as an alcohol-related violent act, will in many cases have more than one level of cause. The most obvious consequences of alcohol are clearly pharmacological in nature: psychomotor disturbances in the form of staggering, slurred speech, an unsteady look, and cognitive effects manifested as attentional and perceptual impairment as well as irregularities in thought processes. Social beliefs regarding alcohol effects will, in addition, determine the outcome of an alcohol-associated social event. The cultural symbolism attached to alcohol, drinking and intoxication will interact with the other types of factor.

Another complication is that alcohol is not a unitary variable. Pharmaco-biological dose-response curves show relations between levels of blood alcohol and the probability of certain consequences. Biological responses are approximately the same for beer, wine and spirits. In relation to psychosocial effects, however, different forms of alcohol – types of beverage, for example – produce different types of consequence. The few studies that have been carried out indicate that beer, wine and spirits have different risks of being related to aggression. These beverages have different cultural meanings, which affect their consequences in the life of a society. What from a biological point of view is a ratio, or at least an ordinal scale variable (amount of alcohol consumed or level of alcohol in the blood), is in relation to social effects a nominal (categorical) level variable.[6] The social consequences are *alcohol-related* but the relationship is located in the culture or, more basically, in the minds of participating individuals and in the (in part culturally determined) cues available in the immediate

---

[6] Beverages may differ as regards bioavailability. Even different types of distilled spirits and wine brands differ as to type and amount of congeners. There is no systematic evidence, however, that these would cause differences in behaviour in addition to the effects of blood alcohol levels.

situation; the relationship is not in the physiological state of the drinker's organism.

Natural-science aspects of alcohol consumption have social relevance and enter into the symbolic meanings of alcohol and drinking in a society. The psychomotor effects of alcohol have social consequences in the form of, for instance, increased risks of accidents and injuries. They also, however, provide signs that are used for ascribing degree of intoxication, behaviour tendencies, moral status, etc. to a person. The meanings given to signs of intoxication depend on the social context in which they are displayed; they invoke very different attributions and lead to different types of reaction in different social contexts.

Alcohol consumption is related to both positive and negative social experiences or occurrences. It is important, however, to specify the kind of 'relatedness': a statistical association, a risk relationship or a causal relationship.

Alcohol can act as a cause on several level types of determination. Pharmacological causality is easiest to prove or disprove, and there is a tendency to limit the term 'cause' to this type of natural-science causality. It is evident, however, from the research carried out so far that alcohol has causal effects in several spheres outside the natural-science sphere, such as the psychological, societal, social-interactional and cultural.

Studies of different cultures indicate that the same type of consumption may have very different outcomes. Fairly large differences are evident even among industrialized societies in Europe. Psychological experiments have shown that people's beliefs about alcohol and its effects determine behaviour under the influence of alcohol. Similar experiments have shown the importance of situational factors, setting and social context in determining the social consequences of drinking.

A convenient way to comprehend the variety of ways in which alcohol consumption can have social consequences is to contrast prevailing social conditions with those that would characterize a totally alcohol-free society.

Even the most directly psychomotor effects of alcohol have symbolic and interactional consequences. A person who is staggering and whose speech is slurred, and is apparently under the influence of alcohol, will meet with specific types of behaviour expressing attitudes and beliefs about drunken persons in the social environment. This type of alcohol-related effect is clearly manifested in response to behaviour that appears to be an effect of alcohol intoxication but in fact has a different cause, such as a neurological disorder.

What from the point of view of one field of inquiry is based on mere chance or a spurious relationship may be a substantive and interesting relationship viewed from another field of inquiry. If only the pharmacologically determined effects of alcohol use are to be considered as being truly caused by alcohol, the other effects become lodged in the category of mere chance or spuriousness.

Cultures and subcultures differ greatly in the types of behaviour, ritual and social consequence associated with drinking. The differences can to some extent be predicted from the amounts of alcohol consumed in a population and the distribution of individuals with different levels of blood-alcohol-concentration. There is still, however, a considerable residue of unexplained differences, which are likely to be attributable to psychological, social, cultural and situational factors.

REFERENCES

1. Single, E., Collins, D., Easton, B., Harwood, H., Lapsley, H. and Maynard, A. (1996) *International Guidelines for Estimating the Social Costs of Substance Abuse*, Canadian Centre on Substance Abuse, Toronto.
2. MacAndrew, C. and Edgerton, R.B. (1969) *Drunken Comportment*, Aldine, Chicago.
3. Pernanen, K. (1991) *Alcohol in Human Violence*, Guilford Press, New York.
4. Roizen, J. (1993) Issues in the epidemiology of alcohol and violence, in *Alcohol and Interpersonal Violence: Fostering Multidisciplinary Perspectives*, (ed. S. Martin) Washington DC, US Department of Health and Human Services, National Institute on Alcohol Abuse and Alcoholism, (Research Monograph 24).
5. Cherpitel, C.J. (1995) Alcohol and injury in the general population: data from two household samples. *Journal of Studies on Alcohol* 56, 83–89.
6. Lenke, L. (1989) *Alcohol and Criminal Violence: Time Series Analyses in a Comparative Perspective*, Akademitryck, Edsbruk.
7. Takala, H. (1973) Alkoholstrejkens inverkan på uppdagad brottslighet. [The effects of the alcohol strike on detected crimes], *Alkoholpolitik* 36, 14–16.
8. Karaharju, E.O. and Stjernvall, L. (1974) The alcohol factor in accidents. *Injury* 6, 67–79.
9. Bushman, B.J. and Cooper, H.M. (1990) Effects of alcohol on human aggression: an integrative research review. *Psychological Bulletin* 107, 341–354.
10. Hull, J.G. and Bond, C.F. (1986) Social and behavioral consequences of alcohol consumption and expectancy: a meta-analysis. *Psychological Bulletin* 99, 347–360.
11. Marshall, M. (1983) 'Four hundred rabbits': an anthropological view of ethanol as a disinhibitor, in *Alcohol and Disinhibition: Nature and Meaning of the Link* (eds R. Room and G. Collins), Rockville, MD, US Department of Health and Human Services, pp. 186–204.
12. Pernanen, K. (1976) Alcohol and crimes of violence, in *The Biology of Alcoholism: Vol 4 Social Aspects of Alcoholism* (eds B. Kissin and H. Begleiter), Plenum Press, New York, pp. 351–444.

Chapter three

Alcohol consumption and social harm: quantitative research methodology

G. Gmel and E. Gutjahr

This chapter highlights methodological shortcomings of quantitative research into the association of alcohol consumption and social harm. It is organized according to the four key areas of epidemiological research: assessment/measurement (a) of outcome, (b) of exposure, and (c) of covariates, and study design [1, 2]; it considers also several less known designs of research into alcohol-related social harm, and indicates some future research directions.

The main argument is centred on two aspects:

- Research into the association between alcohol consumption and social consequences has to take account of cultural factors.

- Owing to the complexity of dimensions of social harm (= outcome) and alcohol consumption (= exposure), and of their interrelatedness (see Chapter 1), no single design can be optimal for investigating all of them. For example, temporality (that a cause precedes an effect) is a *sine qua non* of causality [2] (a more detailed discussion of causality issues is given in Chapter 2) and is probably best investigated with a cohort design. Commonly with such a design, alcohol consumption is assessed at baseline and outcomes are followed up for from 5 to 15 years [3]. Such a design, we argue, can be used for analysing relationships between only some long-term disease outcomes and volume of drinking, and even for these relationships strict assumptions must be met [4]. There is striking

Harald Klingemann and Gerhard Gmel (eds.), Mapping the Social Consequences of Alcohol Consumption, 33–52.
© *2001 Kluwer Academic Publishers. Printed in Great Britain.*

evidence, however, that drinking pattern (e.g. regular consumption of small quantities regularly or of large quantities on a single occasion) is at least as valid as total volume as a predictor of social consequences [5–11]. Moreover, for certain acute consequences such as accidents or aggression, single-occasion use may be more determinant than long-term use, and therefore study designs other than long-term follow-up may be more appropriate.

A methodological background is set out that may help in interpreting evidence presented in subsequent chapters. Given, however, that scientific evidence accumulates over different kinds of research design (experiments, case-control studies, cohort studies, ecological studies, etc.; see Chapter 2 for an example), weaknesses in any particular design need not prevent its strengths from contributing significantly to knowledge of alcohol-related harm. Similarly, notwithstanding the emphasis here on quantitative research methods and the quantification of social harm, qualitative research may be an even more useful means of investigating the etiology and mechanisms of alcohol-related social harm [12].

ASSESSMENT OF OUTCOME

It is a tenet of epidemiological research that '[t]he outcome disorder under study should be well-defined and the included cases should be adequately validated from original clinical records' [1, p. 1768]. As, however, much of the research on social harm relies on self-reported information, this section, on outcome assessment, is concerned with data derived from self-reporting.

Table 1 gives examples of questions and statements commonly used in surveys for assessing social harm; most social-harm items are in the tradition of the problem-drinking items used in the early surveys of the Alcohol Research Group at Berkeley [13].

The use of such items for outcome assessment of social harm raises a number of issues. Usually, different items are combined in a scale. Following the clinimetrical [21] approach, a standard way is the 'at least one out of ...' [17, 22] measure; another is the adding up of items [11, 16]. The clinimetrical approach may be criticized on at least three grounds: (a) it indicates mainly the occurrence of problems and not their severity or frequency; (b) it attaches to all problems the same weight of severity; and (c) it combines outcomes that are associated with different patterns of exposure. As Skog [23], for instance, has argued, a positive correlation of severity of problems with consumption would exaggerate the contribution of light and moderate drinkers to the overall social-harm score. An affirmative answer to a question on whether a respondent had experienced a drink-related problem would carry the same weight whether the problem was trivial or severe or, as Heath has more cogently observed, unless severity is measured, headache, for example, would be equated with 'vehicular homicide' [24].

Social-harm scales have rarely been psychometrically tested – i.e. analysed as to whether (a) different items can be subsumed under one factor, and (b) all items load equally strongly for the same factor (technically: constructing a parallel model), which are necessary conditions for aggregating items [11, 18]. Most of these scales, moreover, combine long-term (e.g. financial) with acute (e.g. accidents) consequences. The association between the summary scale and different aspects of exposure (cumulative or maximum) may be blurred.

A second concern about questions such as those set out in Table 1 is that outcome is not assessed independently of exposure. An epidemiological researcher is unlikely to ask 'have you ever had gastritis due to your alcohol consumption'. Recall bias and therefore differential misclassification may result from a respondent who has had an alcohol-related accident recalling exposure (e.g. binge drinking) better than one who has not [2], because of putting more 'effort after meaning' [25] in trying to recall a drinking occasion.

The difficulties are further complicated by such questions as 'Have you lost a job or hurt chances for promotion and raises?', for here even the direction of an effect is determined. Such questions do not take account of potential benefits of alcohol, yet there is ample evidence in the literature of a positive association between drinking and income [26, 27].

Lastly, questions about alcohol-related social consequences often use different time-frames for different consequences (lifetime and past 12 month [28], see also Table 1). At the same time, consumption is usually measured only in a single time-frame, often the past 12 months, and only once (either at baseline in follow-up studies or current in cross-sectional surveys). This gives rise to several complications. First, in a summary measure, consequences that occurred in different periods of life are aggregated and may not, therefore, be related to consumption at the time of measurement of consumption. In prospective longitudinal research with measurement of consumption at baseline and assessment of consequences later in time, several assumptions must hold for a potential association between the two to be valid. For long-term consequences this implies that consumption has been stable over the period between assessment of consumption and occurrence of a consequence, and for acute consequences that the consumption reported at the time of interview is indicative of that at the time of the consequences. It is essential also, of course, to know accurately when an outcome occurred since, obviously, consumption (exposure) must precede outcome to invoke a causal inference [1].

It is assumed that all instruments for measuring exposure can measure total volume in a shorter time-span with sufficient reliability and validity, but see Dawson [29] and related comments of Midanik *et al.* [30]. Nutritional epidemiology has established that the measurement of amount of alcohol consumption with food frequency questionnaires (FFQ), an extended version of the QF method, commonly shows higher validity and reliability than measurements of intake of other nutrients (see, for example, results from European Investigation into Cancer and Nutrition [31–33]).

Table 1 Examples of questions and statements used to measure social consequences

Herd [14]	Schuckit et al. [15]	Burton and Williamson, Single, Rehm et al. [16–18]	Bailey [19]	Midanik [20]
Job problems, problems with fulfilling major obligations – I have lost a job or nearly lost one, because of drinking – Drinking may have hurt my chance for promotion, or raises, or better jobs – Was there ever a time when you felt that your drinking had harmful effects on your work and employment opportunities?	– Problems at work, school related to drinking – Drinking interfered with work or other obligations – Decreased important activities to drink	– Was there ever a time that you felt alcohol use had a harmful effect on your work, studies or employment opportunities?	– How many times have you come to school drunk?	– Lost or nearly lost a job because of drinking – People at work suggested I should cut down on drinking – Drinking hurt chances of promotion and raises
Police problems – I had trouble with the law about drinking when driving was not involved – I have been arrested for driving after drinking – A policeman warned or questioned me because of my drinking	– Arrest for alcohol-related behavior (not DWI) – Arrested for drinking driving (DWI)	– Contact with the police due to drinking	– In the past 12 months, how many times have you driven a car after drinking? – In the past 12 months, how many times has your drinking caused problems with the police?	– In relation to alcohol, questioned or warned by a police officer – Been in trouble with the law – Arrests

Table 1 (cont.)

Herd [14]	Schuckit et al. [15]	Burton and Williamson. Single. Rehm et al. [16–18]	Bailey [19]	Midanik [20]
Health problems				
– I had an illness connected with drinking, which kept me from working or my regular activities for a week or more – A physician suggested I could cut down on drinking – I felt my drinking was becoming a serious threat to my physical health – Was there ever a time when you felt that your drinking had harmful effects on your health?	– Psychological impairment related to drinking	– Physical health; negative effects on health (due to drinking); negative effects on happiness or outlook on life (due to drinking)		– Drinking becoming a serious threat to physical health – Physicians suggesting cutting down on drinking
Accidents				
– My drinking contributed to getting hurt in an accident in a car or elsewhere – My drinking contributed to getting involved in an accident in which someone else was hurt or property, such as an auto, was damaged	– Accidental self-injury while intoxicated – Driving accident due to drinking – Drinking/drunk while in hazardous situations		– In the past 12 months, how many times have you gotten into an accident or gotten hurt while drinking?	– Getting involved in an accident – Getting hurt in an accident

Table 1 (cont.)

Herd [14]	Schuckit et al. [15]	Burton and Williamson, Single, Rehm et al. [16–18]	Bailey [19]	Midanik [20]
Belligerence - I have gotten into a fight while drinking - I have gotten into a heated argument while drinking	- Physical fights while intoxicated - Hit or threw things while drinking - Arguments while drinking - Hitting others without fighting while intoxicated			- Alcohol-related heated arguments - Alcohol-related fights
Financial problems - Was there ever a time when you felt that your drinking had a harmful effect on your financial position?		- Negative effect on one's financial position		
Problems with spouse, relatives or friends - Did your spouse's feelings about your drinking break up your relationship with him/her or threaten to break it up - A spouse or someone I lived with threatend to leave me because of my drinking - A spouse or someone I lived with became angry about my drinking or the way I behaved while drinking	- Hit a family member while drinking - Problems with family, friend due to drinking - Lost friends due to drinking - Drinking caused problems in love relationship - Objections about drinking from family/friends/MD	- Problems with friendship and social life (due to drinking) - Negative effects on home and family life	- In the past 12 months how many times has your drinking caused problems with your friends? - In the past 12 months how many times has your drinking caused problems with your parents/family?	- Spouse or someone lived with got angry - Spouse or someone lived with threatened to leave

Table 1 (cont.)

Herd [14]	Schuckit et al. [15]	Burton and Williamson, Single, Rehm et al. [16–18]	Bailey [19]	Midanik [20]
– Was there ever a time when you felt that your drinking had a harmful effect on your home life or marriage? – Did your spouse or someone you lived with ever feel that you should drink less or act differently when you drank? – Did your mother's (father's, other relatives') feelings about your drinking threaten to break up your relationship with her? – Did your mother (father, other relatives) ever feel that you should drink less or act differently when you drank? – Did a girlfriend's or boyfriend's (any other friend's) feelings about your drinking break up your relationship with him/her or threaten to break it up? – Did your girlfriend or boyfriend (any other friend) ever feel that you should drink less or act differently when you drank?				

Future studies are unlikely to use prospective designs with multiple measurement/assessment points. Hence, whenever the design must cover long time-frames (because of either a long induction period or a low incidence of outcomes) [29], studies must rely on retrospective, self-reported information. It must be possible, therefore, with the instruments used (questionnaires, structured interviews, etc.) to collect consumption data of different phases of drinking across a long time span (periods of high and low drinking), and also to determine accurately the time of these different drinking periods as well as the time of the occurrence of different consequences. Instruments should be able to obtain answers to the following questions, for example: *When was it exactly that you had the accident? How much had you drunk when you had the accident? When was it exactly that you drank the most? How much did you drink at the time when you drank most?* More research is needed to determine the accuracy of recall of those time-points and their associated exposure and outcomes.

ASSESSMENT OF EXPOSURE

'The drug exposure that is under study should be well-defined in terms of timing, dose, and duration of use' [1, p. 1768]. However, '... recorded information on exposure is not often available' [2, p. 141]. Researchers, therefore, usually have to rely on data derived from self-reporting, which are prone to such distortions as underreporting, social desirability, or recall bias. For this reason also, this section is concerned with data derived from self-reporting.

Currently used instruments for assessing self-reported consumption concentrate upon volume of drinking in a very narrowly specified period of time (a week, a month, three months, 12 months). The most often used are the quantity-frequency (QF) and the graduated-frequency (GF) instruments or weekly diaries (WD) [34–36]. QF-measures, the results of multiplying 'usual' frequencies by 'usual' quantities per occasion, are almost exclusively applicable to average consumption and cumulative exposure. Diaries, which are more flexible with regard to variability of drinking, usually have very restricted time-frames (e.g. one week) and may therefore misclassify infrequent drinkers or overlook heavy drinking occasions [37].

If data on consumption are being collected to examine its association with social consequences, however, volume of drinking in a narrow time-span alone may be insufficient: variability of drinking and maximum exposure are at least of equal value. In addition, as Dawson [29] has pointed out, many social consequences are so rare that their incidence can only be determined reliably over a relatively long time-frame. Exposure must also be measured over a long period, therefore. As Polich *et al.* [38] have pointed out, especially for high-risk drinkers, the dominant pattern of behaviour of drinkers over time is change. Research in general populations has confirmed this lack of stability in drinking pattern over the life-course [25, 39–41]. The assessment of alcohol consumption at a single time-point, covering only a short time-span of consumption, may fail, therefore, to represent accurately the consumption pattern associated with the consequence. There has, regrettably, been little research to develop and standardize instruments for measuring variations in drinking pattern over periods of more than one week or 12 months. Current research suggests that instruments commonly employed for assessing alcohol consumption over longer periods are of questionable use. Standard assessment instruments, such as food frequency questionnaires, have lower validity for irregular than for regular drinkers [42], and reproducibility decreases with the time-span for which intake needs to be measured [43].

Instruments for measuring maximum exposure (e.g. drinking to intoxication, bingeing, occasional heavy intake) have similar, or even more serious, shortcomings; those most often used are the so-called 5+ (or 8+, or 12+) – the consumption of five drinks or more on one occasion or during a day [14, 44–46]. In addition, although the 5+ measure has been used over almost 40 years of alcohol research, its inherent meaning (is 5+ during a day enough to make one drunk?) or its empirical foundation is still to be discovered [20]. Other measures of binge drinking or heavier episodic drinking include 'drinking enough to feel drunk (or intoxicated)', 'to feel the effects', or 'to feel high' [20], two days of intoxication [47] or drinking half of the recommended weekly consumption in a single setting [48]. Of course, the wording of items, such as 'feeling the effects' or even 'intoxication', often presented to respondents without any descriptive term for the item leaves a wide range for subjective interpretation of its meaning, and may vary widely among individuals [49].

COVARIATES: CONFOUNDING AND CONTROL VARIABLES

In accordance with epidemiological principles, the relationship between social harm and alcohol use must be controlled for variables that may confound, mediate, or moderate the association – so-called third variables. They include sociodemographic characteristics (e.g. sex, age, socioeconomic status) and variables related with drinking, e.g. time of day when drinking occurs [50], or week-end rather than work-day drinking [51], location, setting and social context such as at home or in bars [52–54]. One third-variable, however, is often overlooked or difficult to assess, namely the culture-specific norms and expectancies about drinking and ideas of what constitutes social harm [24, 55]. These culture-dependent norms and expectancies about the association of alcohol consumption and harm also influence the interpretation of questionnaire items about alcohol-related harm. Rehm and Fischer [56] have emphasized that harm items often measure attitudes about harm as well as harm *per se*. They illustrate this by an extreme example, that of vomiting into a neighbour's garden during a party, which may not be seen as social harm in a wet culture such as Bavaria's, but certainly would in other cultures. Accordingly, the 'time out' hypothesis states that drunken behaviour is influenced more by norms about what it should be than by the pharmacological effect of alcohol [57]. Cross-cultural research has shown that it is difficult to adapt drinking norms of 'wet' cultures to 'dry' cultures, that norms related to drinking and drunkenness vary widely across cultures, and that the association between drinking and reporting of consequences may, therefore, also vary [58–60].

STUDY DESIGN

So far we have argued that analysis of alcohol consumption and social harm is complicated by at least the following points:

- Exposure must be defined in terms of average (and/or cumulative) as well as maximum exposure
- Outcomes are rarely defined objectively and questionnaires usually measure, besides actual social harm, attitudes toward what is perceived as social harm
- Social consequences and their association with drinking vary with the length of the interval between the manifestation of a drinking pattern and onset of outcome, namely intervals that are relatively short for acute, and longer for long-term, consequences; both time-points must be determined with precision, as must consumption at both time-points as well as during the period between them
- Many social consequences are culture-bound, and hence it may not be possible with studies within a single culture to examine the impact of culture-specific factors.

The study design must, consequently, match the theoretical association between exposure pattern and type of outcome. In this chapter some of the shortcomings of classical epidemiological designs (cohort studies, case-control studies, cross-sectional studies, experiments) in relation to certain social consequences are discussed. Every design has its strengths, of course, and may be optimal in connection with other social consequences. Experimental designs have their place in the laboratory for investigating, for example, the aggravating effect of alcohol consumption on level of aggressiveness [overview, e.g. 61, 62] and on reactivity and driving ability [63–65, p. 1015], or the impact of expectancies of the effects of alcohol consumption (see, e.g. the meta-analytic review of McKay and Schare [66]). Such designs have limited use in the 'real world', however, where social interaction, level of intoxication, and cultural influences are crucial variables.

A serious shortcoming of most long-term cohort-studies is that alcohol exposure is measured at baseline only and, therefore, often long before the consequences are measured. Variability in drinking and drinking pattern is often not well reflected in baseline measurement of consumption, which in itself may not be indicative of consumption pattern at the time of onset of a disease or a social consequence or at the time of an event. For example, a long-term prospective design with assessment of average intake at baseline is probably not the best for investigating outcomes that are related with drinking in the event (e.g. at the time of violent behaviour or an accident).

Case-control studies often use emergency-room data or police records. Emergency-room studies have disadvantages: there is generally no satisfactory control group; there is liable to be a bias towards increasing severity of incidents; the interval between occurrence of an incident and assessment of alcohol consumption is typically short (e.g. the more severe the incident, the sooner the individual is likely to arrive); and blood may not be sampled because of severity of an incident and consequent threat to life [12, 67–69]. Police and court records have similar disadvantages. They may not represent an unbiased sample of all violent incidents, as only a small part of violent behaviour comes to police attention [70]. Even if the sample were representative, however, blood or breath tests, for example, would give only an indication of an association between alcohol and an event, given that it is impossible to determine how many such accidents or violent acts would have happened even without any drinking. As Room [55, p. 380] has stated about traffic accidents: 'this indeterminacy is overridden, for instance, when an alcohol cause is assigned in the statistics to a crash whenever a driver has been drinking'.

Cross-sectional surveys are limited because of recall bias and assessment of causality, for example. They can show a strong association between post-traumatic stress disorder and alcohol use, for instance, but longitudinal research usually shows a causal path from injury, rape or other violent behaviour to, rather than from, increased alcohol consumption.

The influence of cultural factors varies across cultures or regions and is usually analysed by ecological studies – for example, correlational studies of aggregate-level data of alcohol consumption and outcomes across different cultures or regions [71]. Time-series analysis is also of the ecological type [72]. A defect of such studies is the so-called ecological fallacy or ecological bias. Technically, this means that information on the joint distribution of variables is missing. Practically, it means that effects identified by ecological studies may not hold, or may even be contrary to effects, at the individual level. Ecological analysis may show higher suicide rates in a particular religious group than in other groups. This group, however, may be a religious minority living in the area under study, and its minority status rather than its religion may be the reason for committing suicide. This would be an effect of interaction between religion and the religious composition of the area of residence [72], which has not been controlled for in the ecological analysis. Of course, in ecological analysis it is usually impossible to control for all third variables.

SOME LESS-KNOWN DESIGNS FOR INVESTIGATION OF ALCOHOL-RELATED SOCIAL HARM

Other designs, mainly extensions of those discussed above, also have weaknesses, and are, therefore, not 'better' or more universally applicable than those described above. Some, however, though seldom used, have certain advantages, and may increase our understanding of alcohol-related consequences. They include nested case-control studies, pseudo-panel studies, multi-level analysis, roadside surveys, and at-scene studies.

Nested case-control studies

As has been seen above, the accuracy of the assessment of risk of social harm from drinking is determined largely by the length of the interval between consumption and outcome events as well as by variability of exposure over time. One way to reduce measurement errors such as recall bias or unmeasured changes in consumption may be to increase the number of measurement points (interviews) and reduce the interval between them. The limitations of such a design are clear [73]: multiple time-measures are extremely costly in both time and resources; and problem drinkers can be very difficult to follow up; this difficulty increases with length of follow-up and number of measurement points, with consequent serious attrition bias. The innovative touch-tone telephone method [74–76] may increase compliance and reduce the cost of such a design.

Nested case-control studies or case-cohort studies [2] are one way of reducing cost. A cohort may be followed up by relatively inexpensive screening or with information readably available from records. Within the cohort, it may be possible to conduct more efficient case-control studies in which the control series is selected by random sampling from the non-cases of the cohort.

Pseudo-panel studies

A second possibility is the pseudo-panel approach [73], so called as it consists of a retrospective cross-sectional study in which questions are asked in 'pseudo-panel' form, namely time-series questions asked separately, as though the interviews were separated by time periods. Prospective studies using multiple time-measurements are more reliable than retrospective measurements [77], but reliability of retrospective studies can be improved by pseudo-panel questions. A Japanese study by Takatsuka *et al.* [78] has shown that the pseudo-panel approach can be useful: over a period of nine years, differences between past and current measures of food intake, including alcohol, were higher than differences between past measures and the nine-year recall of past intake. This suggests that recall measures of intake are preferable for assessing past consumption to equating current with past consumption. Similar results have been found with shorter time lags [79]. Clearly, the improvement of retrospective methods depends heavily on the development of instruments for assessing consumption over the lifetime. A growing body of research is indicating that lifetime drinking history may be measured with 'reasonable' validity and reliability ([25] for a review of the discussion surrounding lifetime drinking histories at the International Workshop on Consumption Measures and Models for Use in Policy Developments and Evaluation, held in Bethesda in May 1997 [80–82]) even when questions are administered by telephone or computer [83].

Multi-level analysis

There is much evidence that the relationship between alcohol consumption and consequences is not cross-culturally stable. Any cross-cultural investigation into these relationships, therefore, must take account of cultural norms and patterns of drinking, but also of provisions of alcohol policy in relation to, for example, traffic regulations or penalties for public drunkenness. The most common analysis of cross-cultural differences is of the 'ecological analysis' type and is, therefore, prone to ecological bias and insufficient controlling for confounding at the individual level. A powerful method of analysing individual-level data as well as ecological or contextual effects is multilevel analysis [84, 85]. It permits the analysis of hierarchically structured data. This structure occurs, for instance, if a study includes people from different countries. Then individuals in one country are exposed to the same set of conditions (the same law enforcement, the same legal blood-alcohol-concentration limits, the same opening-hours etc.) but differ from people in other countries in these respects. Thus, individual-level relationships are clustered within aggregate-level characteristics. Aggregate-level variables could be, for example, sales data, percentages of abstainers, average number of drinking days, legal blood-alcohol-concentration levels [86].

Such an analysis could be used to examine not only how the risks of social consequences such as aggression, or driving under the influence of alcohol, are related to volume and patterns of drinking, but also whether this relationship varies across cultures and what variables at the aggregate level explain such a variation.

Roadside surveys

Much of the information about alcohol involvement in social harm, especially on casualties of traffic accidents, violent acts, etc., comes from case-control studies (including emergency-room studies). The most common shortcoming of such studies concerns the choice of a suitable control group. To correctly assess a control group the following points should be respected [1, 2]:

- The time a subject is eligible to become a control should also be the time the subject is eligible to become a case.

- Each case in a case-control study should have been eligible to be a control before the occurrence of the event or disorder; each control should be eligible to become a case at the time of occurrence of the event or disorder disease onset.

- When comparability is achieved, the risk of developing the disorder or being involved in an accident, for instance, is the same for people exposed to alcohol and those unexposed – unless alcohol is associated with the outcome disorder.

These conditions are often not well applied either in emergency-room studies (e.g. alcohol consumption is also higher in emergency patients chosen as controls than in the general population) or in studies for which the general population is chosen as control sample (e.g. in driver-accident studies controls should be drivers; controls are not at risk of bar aggression if they do not visit bars or at least not when bar aggression usually occurs).

For traffic accidents there is a valuable though rarely used study-design alternative: roadside surveys. Probably the best known study of this kind was conducted by Borkenstein and colleagues [87, 88, but see 89 for methodological flaws in original analysis]. For a roadside survey, a random sample of drivers is drawn and their blood-alcohol concentration is measured. If the sample is adequately representative of the geographical area and of the time-span in which cases were selected, it can be used as a control series – i.e. the excess risk of drivers under the influence can be calculated because the percentage of accident-free drivers with a given blood-alcohol concentration can be estimated from the control series. Recently, Krüger [90] estimated for Germany that 10.8% of all accidents were alcohol-related, whereas the percentage of accidents involving drivers with testable blood-alcohol concentration (>0.02%) was 16.8% and that involving drivers with a concentration of 0.08% was 12.3%. Hence, the legal limit of 0.08% as an indicator of alcohol-relatedness would overestimate the proportion of accidents attributable to alcohol.

The 'at-scene' study

A different study design that can be used to ensure an adequate control series is the so-called 'at-scene' study. It permits the collection of cases and controls directly at the time and location of an event (in bars, on the road, etc.), namely at the scene. Its advantages are straightforward: controls interviewed at the scene have the same situational factors as the cases (weather conditions, loudness, etc.). It is very expensive, however, and may lack representativeness owing to, for example, limited geographical coverage of the study [91]. An alert system must be established and the research team must arrive immediately after the event. This study type may add valuable information, however. In Memphis, Tenn., for example, a research team accompanying police on calls for domestic assaults – a particular form of at-scene study [92] – found that most victims who had called the police used medical facilities rarely, which suggests that, as regards domestic violence, samples used for emergency-room studies may be selective.

CONCLUSIONS

The conclusions resulting from consideration of assessment/measurement of outcome, exposure, and covariates, and of study design indicate that future research into alcohol consumption and social harm should be guided by the following principles:

The analysis of outcomes should match their association with drinking patterns

For each outcome the theoretical relationship with exposure – i.e. whether average consumption (= volume) or heavy-drinking occasions or both are important – should be defined, and outcomes with different associations with drinking patterns should be analysed separately. Whenever combined scales of multiple outcomes are used for assessment/measurement, their psychometric properties (unidimensionality, weights for each contributory consequence, etc.) must be culture-specifically tested within the context of the analysis (general population, clinical population, etc.).

The development of assessment instruments should focus on patterns of drinking

There is now sufficient evidence that instruments that assess/measure total volume or average volume in a short time period can evince acceptable psychometric properties (reliability, validity, reproducibility). There is an urgent need, however, to determine whether instruments used to assess/measure longer time-frames and patterns of drinking – especially maximum exposure (bingeing) and different exposure periods (phases in life with moderate regular consumption, high regular consumption, abstinence, frequent heavy drinking, etc.) – can evince similarly acceptable properties.

Methods of recall should be improved

Future studies are unlikely to use prospective designs with multiple measurement points. Hence, whenever the design must cover longer time-frames because of either a long induction period or a low incidence of outcomes [29], the study must rely on retrospective self-reported information. Methods need to be developed, therefore, that can assess different phases/periods of drinking as well as determine accurately the time-points of different outcomes. More research is needed to determine the accuracy of retrospective assessment of those time-points and their associated exposure and outcomes.

Research should concentrate on culturally dependent norms, expectancies and attitudes

Current findings on alcohol-related social harm are strongly influenced by cultural factors. Research is needed that elucidates such factors and therefore helps to clarify apparently contradictory findings. This means research that not only detects differences between cultures but also distinguishes between, on the one hand, culturally determined attitudes as indicated by responses and, on the other, actual behaviour that is culturally influenced. Meta-analytic studies and hierarchical linear modelling may help to disentangle cultural variations in the relationships between alcohol consumption and social harm as well as culturally influenced differences in the understanding of what constitutes social harm and in its reporting.

REFERENCES

1. Jick, H. *et al.* (1998) Principles of epidemiological research on adverse and beneficial drug effects. *Lancet* 352, 1767–1770.
2. Rothman, K.J. and Greenland, S. (1998) *Modern Epidemiology*, Lippincott-Raven, Philadelphia, PA.
3. English, D.R. *et al.* (1995) *The Quantification of Drug Caused Morbidity and Mortality in Australia*, Canberra, Commonwealth Department of Human Services and Health.
4. Rehm, J. (2000) Alcohol intake assessment: the facts are even more sobering. *American Journal of Epidemiology* 151, 436–438.
5. Room, R. *et al.* (1995) The risk of harm to oneself from drinking, Canada 1989. *Addiction* 90, 499–513.
6. Midanik, L.T. *et al.* (1996) Risk functions for alcohol-related problems in a 1988 US national sample. *Addiction* 91, 1427–1437.
7. Bondy, S.J. (1996) Overview of studies on drinking patterns and consequences. *Addiction* 91, 1663–1674.
8. Plant, M.A. *et al.*, eds. (1997) *Alcohol: Minimising the Harm: What Works?* Free Association Books, London.
9. Rehm, J. *et al.* (1996) On the emerging paradigm of drinking patterns and their social and health consequences. *Addiction* 91(11), 1615–1621.
10. Grant, M. and Litvak, J., eds. (1998) *Drinking Patterns and Their Consequences*, Taylor and Francis, Washington, DC.
11. Rehm, J. and Gmel, G. (1999) Patterns of alcohol consumption and social consequences. Results from an 8-year follow-up study in Switzerland. *Addiction* 94(6), 899–912.
12. Roizen, J. (1997) Epidemiological issues in alcohol-related violence, in *Recent Developments in Alcoholism* (ed. M. Galanter), Plenum Press, New York/London, pp. 7–37 (13).

13. Cahalan, D. and Room, R. (1974) *Problem Drinking Among American Men*, Rutgers Center of Alcohol Studies, New Brunswick, NJ.
14. Herd, D. (1994) Predicting drinking problems among black and white men: results from a national survey. *Journal of Studies on Alcohol* **55**, 61–71.
15. Schuckit, M.A. *et al.* (1995) The time course of development of alcohol-related problems in men and women. *Journal of Studies on Alcohol* **56**, 218–225.
16. Burton, T.L. and Williamson, D.L. (1995) Harmful effects of drinking and the use and perceived effectiveness of treatment. *Journal of Studies on Alcohol* **56**, 611–615.
17. Single, E. (1994) Implications of potential health benefits of moderate drinking for specific elements of alcohol policy: towards a harm-reduction approach for alcohol. *Contemporary Drug Problems* **21**(2), 275–285.
18. Rehm, J. *et al.* (1999) A reliability and validity analysis of an alcohol-related harm scale for surveys. *Journal of Studies on Alcohol* **60**(2), 203–208.
19. Bailey, S.L. (1999) The measurement of problem drinking in young adulthood. *Journal of Studies on Alcohol* **60**(2), 234–244.
20. Midanik, L.T. (1999) Drunkenness, feeling the effects and 5+ measures. *Addiction* **94**(6), 887–897.
21. Wright, J. and Feinstein, A. (1992) A comparative contrast of clinimetric and psychometric methods for constructing indexes and rating scales. *Journal of Clinical Epidemiology* **45**, 1201–1218.
22. Stockwell, T. *et al.* (1996) Unravelling the preventive paradox for acute alcohol problems. *Drug and Alcohol Review* **15**, 7–5.
23. Skog, O.-J. (1999) The prevention paradox revisited. *Addiction* **94**(5), 751–757.
24. Heath, D.B. (1998) Cultural variations among drinking patterns, in *Drinking Patterns and Their Consequences* (eds M. Grant and J. Litvak), Taylor and Francis, Bristol, PA, pp. 103–128.
25. Lemmens, P.H. (1998) Measuring Lifetime Drinking Histories. *Alcoholism: Clinical and Experimental Research* **22**(2), 29S–36S.
26. Berger, M.C. and Leigh, J.P. (1988) The effect of alcohol use on wages. *Applied Economics* **20**, 1343–1351.
27. Sindelar, J. (1998) Social costs of alcohol. *Journal of Drug Issues* **28**(3), 763–780.
28. Harwood, H.J. *et al.* (1984) *Economic Costs to Society of Alcohol and Drug Abuse and Mental Illness: 1980*, Research Triangle Institute, Research Triangle Park, NC (Report to Alcohol, Drug Abuse, and Mental Health Administration).
29. Dawson, D.A. (1998) Measuring alcohol consumption: limitations and prospects for improvement. *Addiction* **93**(7), 965–968.
30. Midanik, L.T. *et al.* (1998) Comments on Dawson's 'Measuring alcohol consumption: limitations and prospects for improvement'. *Addiction* **93**(7), 969–977.
31. Bohlscheid-Thomas, S. *et al.* (1997) Reproducibility and relative validity of energy and macronutrient intake of a food frequency questionnaire developed for the German part of the EPIC project. European Prospective Investigation into Cancer and Nutrition. *International Journal of Epidemiology* **26**(Suppl 1), S71–S81.
32. Kroke, A. *et al.* (1999) Validation of a self-administered food-frequency questionnaire administered in the European Prospective Investigation into Cancer and Nutrition (EPIC) Study: comparison of energy, protein and macronutrient intakes estimated with the doubly labeled water, urinary nitrogen, and repeated 24-h dietary recall methods. *American Journal of Clinical Nutrition* **70**(4), 439–447.
33. Kaaks, R. *et al.* (1997) Pilot phase studies on the accuracy of dietary intake measurements in the EPIC project: overall evaluation of results. European Prospective Investigation into Cancer and Nutrition. *International Journal of Epidemiology* **26**(Suppl 1), S26–S36.
34. Room, R. (1990) Measuring alcohol consumption in the United States: methods and rationales. *Research Advances in Alcohol and Drug Problems* **10**, 39–80.

35. Rehm, J. (1988) Measuring quantity, frequency, and volume of drinking. *Alcoholism: Clinical and Experimental Research* **22**(2), 4S–14S.
36. Feunekes, G.I.J. et al. (1999) Alcohol intake assessment: the sober facts. *American Journal of Epidemiology* **150**(1), 105–112.
37. Rehm, J. et al. (1999) Assessment methods for alcohol consumption, prevalence of high risk drinking and harm: a sensitivity analysis. *International Journal of Epidemiology* **28**, 219–224.
38. Polich, J.M. et al. (1980) *The Course of Alcoholism: Four Years Later*, Rand Corporation, Santa Monica.
39. Johnstone, B.M. et al. (1996) Determinants of life-course variation in the frequency of alcohol consumption: meta-analysis of studies from the collaborative alcohol-related longitudinal project. *Journal of Studies on Alcohol* **57**(5), 494–506.
40. Lemmens, P.H. et al. (1997) Measurement of lifetime exposure to alcohol: data quality of a self-administered questionnaire and impact on risk assessment. *Contemporary Drug Problems* **24**, 581–600.
41. Johnson, F.W. et al. (1998) Drinking over the life course within gender and ethnic groups: a hyperparametric analysis. *Journal of Studies on Alcohol* **59**(5), 568–580.
42. Ferraroni, M. et al. (1996) Validity and reproducibility of alcohol consumption in Italy. *International Journal of Epidemiology* **25**(4), 775–782.
43. Lowik, M.R. et al. (1999) Dependence of dietary intake estimates on the time frame of assessment. *Regulatory Toxicology and Pharmacology* **30**(2 Pt 2), S48–S56.
44. Wechsler, H. et al. (1994) Health and behavioural consequences of binge drinking in college – a national survey of students at 140 campuses. *Journal of the American Medical Association* **272**, 1671–1677.
45. Knupfer, G. (1984) The risks of drunkenness (or, ebrietas resurrecta). A comparison of frequent intoxication indices and of population sub-groups as to problem risks. *British Journal of Addiction* **79**(2), 185–196.
46. Conigrave, K.M. et al. (1995) Predictive capacity of the AUDIT questionnaire for alcohol-related harm. *Addiction* 90(11), 1479–1485.
47. Schuckit, M.A. et al. (1993) Clinical course of alcoholism in 636 male inpatients. *American Journal of Psychiatry* **150**, 786–792.
48. Norman, P. et al. (1998) Understanding binge drinking among young people: an application of the Theory of Planned Behaviour. *Health Education Research* **13**(2), 163–169.
49. Conrod, P.J. et al. (1997) Validation of a measure of excessive drinking: frequency per year that BAL exceeds 0.08%. *Substance Use and Misuse* **32**(5), 587–607.
50. Dawson, D.A. (1996) Temporal drinking patterns and variation in social consequences. *Addiction* **91**(11), 1623–1635.
51. Simpura, J. (1987) *Finnish Drinking Habits: Results from Interview Surveys Held in 1968, 1976 and 1984*, Finnish Foundation for Alcohol Studies, Helsinki.
52. Single, E. and Wortley, S. (1993) Drinking in various settings as it relates to demographic variables and level of consumption: findings from a national survey in Canada. *Journal of Studies on Alcohol* **54**, 590–599.
53. Knibbe, R. (1998) Measuring Drinking Context. *Alcoholism: Clinical and Experimental Research* **22**(2), 15S–20S.
54. Rossow, I. (1996) Alcohol-related violence: the impact of drinking pattern and drinking context. *Addiction* **91**(11), 1651–1661.
55. Room, R. (1996) Alcohol consumption and social harm – conceptual issues and historical perspectives. *Contemporary Drug Problems* **23**, 373–388.
56. Rehm, J. and Fischer, B. (1997) Measuring harm: implications for alcohol epidemiology, in *Alcohol: Minimising the Harm: What Works?* (eds M.A. Plant et al., eds), Free Association Books, London, pp. 248–261.

57. Kallmen, H. and Gustafson, R. (1998) Alcohol and disinhibition. *European Addiction Research* **4**(4), 150–162.
58. Gureje, O. *et al.* (1997) Problems related to alcohol use: a cross-cultural perspective. *Culture, Medicine and Psychiatry* **21**(2), 199–211.
59. Schmidt, L. and Room, R. (1999) Cross-cultural applicability in international classifications and research on alcohol dependence. *Journal of Studies on Alcohol* **60**(4), 448–462.
60. Bloomfield, K. *et al.* (1999) *Alcohol Consumption and Alcohol Problems among Women in European Countries*, Berlin, Institute for Medical Informatics, Biostatistics and Epidemiology, Free University of Berlin (Project Final Report).
61. Graham, K. *et al.* (1996) Circumstances when drinking leads to aggression: an overview of research findings. *Contemporary Drug Problems* **23**, 493–557.
62. Graham, K. *et al.* (1998) Current directions in research on understanding and preventing intoxicated aggression. *Addiction* **93**(5), 659–676.
63. Moskowitz, H. and Robinson, C. (1988) *Effects of Low Doses of Alcohol on Driving-Related Skills: A Review of the Evidence*, US Department of Transportation, Washington, DC.
64. Krüger, H.P. *et al.*, eds. (1993) *Alcohol, Drugs and Traffic Safety – T'92*. Verlag TÜV Rheinland, Cologne, Germany (Effects of low alcohol dosages: a review of the literature), pp. 763–778.
65. Eckhardt, M.J. *et al.* (1998) Effects of moderate alcohol consumption on the central nervous system. *Alcoholism: Clinical and Experimental Research* **22**, 998–1040.
66. McKay, D. and Schare, M.L. (1999) The effects of alcohol and alcohol expectancies on subjective reports and physiological reactivity: a meta-analysis. *Addictive Behaviors* **24**(5), 633–647.
67. Voas, R.B. (1993) Issues in cross-national comparisons of crash data. *Addiction* **88**(7), 959–967.
68. Cherpitel, C.J. (1993) Alcohol and injuries: a review of international emergency room studies. *Addiction* **88**(7), 923–937.
69. Borges, G. *et al.* (1998) Male drinking and violence-related injury in the emergency room. *Addiction* **93**(1), 103–112.
70. Pernanen, K. (1991) *Alcohol in Human Violence*, Guilford Press, New York.
71. Colhoun, H. *et al.* (1997) Ecological analysis of collectivity of alcohol consumption in England: importance of average drinker. *British Medical Journal* **314**, 1164–1168.
72. Morgenstern, H. (1998) Ecologic studies, in *Modern Epidemiology* (eds K.J. Rothman and S. Greenland), Lippincott-Raven, Philadelphia, PA, pp. 459–480.
73. Dunham, R.G. (1983) Rethinking the measurement of drinking patterns. *Journal of Studies on Alcohol* **44**(3), 485–493.
74. Mundt, J.C. *et al.* (1995) Cycles of alcohol dependence: frequency-domain analyses of daily drinking logs for matched alcohol-dependent and nondependent subjects. *Journal of Studies on Alcohol* **56**, 491–449.
75. Perrine, M.W. *et al.* (1995) Validation of daily self-reported alcohol consumption using interactive voice response (IVR) technology. *Journal of Studies on Alcohol* **56**, 487–490.
76. Searles, J.S. *et al.* (1995) Self-report of drinking using touch-tone telephone: extending the limits of reliable daily contact. *Journal of Studies on Alcohol* **56**(4), 375–382.
77. Finney, H. (1981) Improving the reliability of retrospective survey measures. *Evaluation Review* **5**(2), 207–229.
78. Takatsuka, N. *et al.* (1996) Validation of recalled food intake in the past in a Japanese population. *Journal of Epidemiology* **6**(1), 9–13.

79. Grant, K.A. *et al.* (1997) Are reconstructed self-reports of drinking reliable. *Addiction* **92**(5), 601–606.
80. Skinner, H.A. and Sheu, W.J. (1982) Reliability of alcohol use indices: the lifetime drinking history and the MAST. *Journal of Studies on Alcohol* **43**, 1157–1170.
81. Sobell, L.C. *et al.* (1988) The reliability of alcohol abusers' self-reports of drinking and life events that occurred in the distant past. *Journal of Studies on Alcohol* **49**, 225–232.
82. McCann, S. *et al.* (1999) Recent alcohol intake as estimated by the Health Habits and History Questionnaire, the Harvard Semiquantitative Food Frequency Questionnaire, and a more detailed Alcohol Intake Questionnaire. *American Journal of Epidemiology* **150**(4), 335–340.
83. Sobell, L.C. *et al.* (1996) The reliability of the alcohol timeline followback when administered by telephone and by computer. *Drug and Alcohol Dependence* **42**(1), 49–54.
84. Bryk, A.S. and Raudenbush, S.W. (1992) *Hierarchical Linear Models*, Sage Publications, Newbury Park.
85. Hox, J.J. (1995) *Applied Multilevel Analysis*, TT-Publikaties, Amsterdam.
86. Rehm, J. and Gmel, G. (2000) Gaps and needs in international alcohol epidemiology. *Journal of Substance Use* **5**, 6–13
87. Borkenstein, R.F. *et al.* (1964) *The Role of the Drinking Driver in Traffic Accidents*, Department of Police Administration, Bloomington, IN.
88. Perrine, M.W. *et al.* (1971) *Alcohol and Highway Safety: Behavioral and Medical Aspects*, National Highway Traffic Safety Administration, Washington, DC (DOT-HS-800-599).
89. Hurst, P.M. *et al.* (1994) The Grand Rapids Dip revisited. *Accident Analysis and Prevention* **26**(5), 647–654.
90. Krüger, H.-P., ed. (1995) *Das Unfallrisiko unter Alkohol: Analyse – Konsequenzen – Massnahme* [Risks of Accidents under the Influence of Alcohol: Analysis – Consequences – Actions], Gustav Fischer Verlag, Stuttgart.
91. Rehm, J. (1993) Methodological approaches and problems in research into alcohol-related accidents and injuries. *Addiction* **88**(7), 885–896.
92. Brookoff, D. *et al.* (1997) Characteristics of participants in domestic violence. Assessment at the scene of domestic assault. *JAMA* **277**(17), 1369–1373.

Chapter four

Consequences of drinking to friends and the close social environment

K. Pernanen

FRIENDS, SOCIAL ENVIRONMENT

Personal relationships are central to constructing human existence. They shape our beliefs, thoughts, acts and identities. Our social institutions are founded on personal relationships and the rules that govern them.

One's social environment consists largely of one's immediate family, other relatives, friends and acquaintances; these often mix and interact, and are sometimes in conflict because of discordant expectancies. Time spent with friends may sometimes reduce time spent with the family, and vice versa. Parents may view suspiciously friends of adolescent offspring, suspecting them of being involved with alcohol or drugs, and thereby influencing their children's habits. Many allusions are made to the conflict between the home and the tavern, between drinking friends and abandoned families. Systematic research on this potential conflict and its resolution is lacking.

Although surprisingly few scientific studies deal directly with the negative or positive impact of drinking on personal relationships outside the family, much of the literature on alcohol use and abuse deals implicitly with the effects of alcohol on relationships with friends. For instance, assessments of social problems associated with alcohol use, and prognoses of improvement or recovery from alcohol abuse, take account of relationships with friends. Some of the most effective interventions in alcohol abuse, such as those based on the philosophy of Alcoholics Anonymous, base their success on support from friends.

Harald Klingemann and Gerhard Gmel (eds.), Mapping the Social Consequences of Alcohol Consumption, 53–65.
© *2001 Kluwer Academic Publishers. Printed in Great Britain.*

There are many more published studies on the reverse influence – how friends and acquaintances affect the drinking patterns of individuals, especially in adolescence. It is in fact difficult to make a clear distinction between the directions of causal influence, since relationships with friends and their links to alcohol use are often part of the same dynamic reciprocal system. Friendships, often hidden under the labels 'peer pressure', 'peer orientations' or 'peer attitudes', affect initiation to alcohol use, and they also influence later drinking patterns and drinking problems [1, 2–5]. Studies have shown that drinking habits in adolescence are reliable predictors of drinking habits and drinking problems later in life [6]. The influence of friendships on an adolescent's drinking, therefore, and the reciprocal influence of the adolescent on the drinking of friends have long-term consequences.

A multiple influence of drinking in relationships with friends is evident in that adolescents, in addition to selecting their friends on the basis of their drinking and other risk-taking behaviour, are influenced also in their drinking behaviour by the new social environment they have chosen [7]. The selection of friends is, therefore, a social consequence of the drinking patterns of the individual, whose drinking is, in turn, affected by them, and whose drinking attitudes and habits form the basis of reception into the friendship circle [8]. Networks of friends and acquaintances have been used to explain the distribution of alcohol consumption in general populations [9].

Friends in the initiation to alcohol use

Initiation to alcohol use often occurs in a group of friends. Peer association determines the age of initiation, the likelihood of continued use and delinquent behaviour related to drinking [10, 11]. Parents are often unaware that their children have been initiated into alcohol use [12]. Family members also act as models for alcohol use, and family influence can offset detrimental influence of peers [4, 13]. Cultural variations in the relative importance of family and friends in the formation of early drinking habits are considerable. In southern Europe, adolescents often drink at meals with the family, at home; in northern Europe they drink much more commonly out-of-doors, clandestinely, with a group of friends or, if at home, while parents are away. In a 1999 survey among Norwegian 15–16-year-old students, a higher proportion reported having taken alcohol most recently in the street or in a park or on the beach than in their own home [14].

The display of risk-taking behaviour is a means of gaining status in a group of adolescents. A social consequence of alcohol use among many adolescents is the respect it commands in a social environment that is, besides the family, their central identity-forming milieu. As risk-taking is a general feature of group interaction among youth, it is difficult to single out the part that alcohol plays in such negative behaviour as violence, unwanted sexual advances, and vandalism. In view, however, of the cognitive impairment due to alcohol, resulting in disregard of consequences, it is likely to play a causal role as one of many features of a risk-taking lifestyle. The symbolic value of drinking itself as a display of risk-taking and rebellion probably differs between cultures.

The 1995 European School Survey Project on Alcohol and Other Drugs was carried out among students aged 15 to 16 years old, in 26 countries [15]. Besides being repeated every few years, this survey has the great advantage of being cross-cultural and focused on an age at which patterns of alcohol use are formed. The in-class questionnaire includes items on problems that the respondents considered were caused by their own drinking. In the 1995 survey, between 8% and 27% of respondents reported that they had experienced such parent relationship problems, and 9–29% problems with friends. Boys in only three of the 26 countries, but girls in 16, reported more such problems with friends than with parents. Criticism of drinking from friends has been found to be more effective among girls than boys, at least in areas with traditional gender-related values [16]. Corcoran and Michels [17] found that 'drinking with friends' was a more negative experience also for adult women than for men. In part, this type of negative experience may be related to unwanted sexual advances towards females, which are relatively common after drinking in groups of friends and acquaintances.

Another question asked was whether respondents had been in a quarrel or argument caused by their own drinking. For 1995, for all countries, the positive responses ranged from 10% to 47% (girls, 9–49%; boys, 12–44%). Between 3% and 28% of respondents reported having been in a scuffle or fight (girls, 2–21%; boys, 3–36%). The widths of these ranges indicate that, in addition to different drinking patterns and typical social contexts of drinking, cultural factors such as the social meaning of drinking occasions may be important in determining the extent to which drinking is linked to aggression and violence and to other consequences for relationships with friends.

Making friends and sustaining friendships through drinking

The effects of drinking on friendships are more situational than are those for family relationships. The latter must endure over time, which makes it harder to escape harmful long-term social effects of alcohol. Relationships between friends may last a long time, but the interaction is less regular, less continuous, and usually less intensive than in the family. There is not the same commitment in time, emotions or finance. Above all, there are not the same responsibilities towards children and other kin. These differences in time perspective and intensity of commitment probably underlie the observed tensions between family and friends with regard to drinking.

One short-term function of drinking outside the family is to meet new people and make new friends. Whether alcohol serves this purpose well has not been sufficiently studied. Many of the positive situational consequences of drinking may be called 'opportunities'. Drinking in the right social context provides extraordinary opportunities for, *inter alia*, enjoyment, camaraderie, 'meeting new people', romance, and sexual relations. The pharmacological effects of alcohol underlying such outcomes are the same as those that give rise to the negative interactional consequences. Some of the psychological effects, such as the narrowing of attentional scope and the related concentration on the 'here-and-now', can explain several outcomes of drinking [18–20]. Among them is the easier and relatively careless interaction that ensues at parties as the participants become more impulsive and spontaneous, and 'open up' and tell more about themselves to complete strangers, for instance. Spontaneity is sought through alcohol – a more immediate link between thought, impulse and action is often the desired outcome of drinking events. These effects of alcohol are used in social occasions to create an intimacy that makes it easy to make friends. The 'time out' or 'bracketing' that characterizes drinking events in many cultures is another feature that promotes spontaneity (see below), as are the strong expectancies of 'disinhibition' that are linked to the use of alcohol.

The alcohol industry in its marketing regularly depicts such opportunities (romantic dinners with wine by candlelight, beer drinking from the bottle in mixed gender groups at summer cottages). In the literature on surveys of alcohol use, drinking-related opportunities are reflected in the types of reason that people give for drinking. Individuals in numerous general-population surveys in many countries have indicated as an important reason that they drink to be sociable or to enhance their social confidence [21]. The alternative reasons presented to the respondent include such items as 'to get along with other people', 'to get courage', and 'to have a good time'. The very term 'social drinker' indicates that for a high proportion of alcohol users convivial drinking with friends and acquaintances is an important factor in decisions on drinking.

Even very young children give social motives as the major reason for intending to drink at a later age [22]. A number of studies indicate that the social nature of drinking is central for several age-groups in a variety of cultures, whether the concept used is 'reasons' for drinking, 'functions' of drinking, or 'expectancies' linked to alcohol. In addition, an increase in amounts consumed at a sitting [23] and problem drinking [24, 25] increase an individual's emphasis on sociability as a reason or expectation linked to drinking.

Drinking events are often used, therefore, as attempts to initiate and sustain bonds between people. An invitation to join a stranger or acquaintance for a drink is in fact an invitation to begin a relationship. Fraternity and university initiations in Europe and the United States are attempts to forge bonds of friendship that also include risk-taking behaviour for status elevation and social acceptance. Risky drinking is a relatively standard feature in these initiations, and deaths and near-deaths from alcohol poisoning and alcohol-related accidents have been reported in recent years [26]. The prevention of 'binge drinking' has consequently become a high priority on university and college campuses in the United States.

Convivial drinking and symbolic acts of solidarity linked to drinking serve as confirmation of friendships. 'Regular' patrons gather in public drinking establishments. Rounds are bought to symbolize common bonds and obligations to the group. The situational nature of behaviour determination under alcohol intoxication aids in this process in the same way as it is a factor in aggravating situational irritants and causing conflict and aggression in other circumstances.

Opportunities created by the ways in which alcohol determines situational behaviour also represent risks. Small-group studies of interaction in drinking groups have been rather few. Data from systematic observations of 660 drinking groups in 28 taverns and bars in a city in Ontario, Canada showed that the level of positive emotional interactions increased steadily as time passed, as did interactions showing negative emotions, such as aggression and depression. At the end of three hours of observation both positive and negative interactions had reached a peak (and may have continued to rise after the conclusion of the observations). Also, fluctuations between positive and negative acts increased as the groups became more intoxicated. Emotionality increases, therefore, in group drinking over time. This can, of course, have both positive and negative consequences.

Friends can also be lost through drinking. Many studies of violent crimes report prevalence figures on the relationships between offender and victim in homicides and assaults. A study in a Canadian city found that 39% of the assailants of respondents in relatively mild cases of alcohol-related violence were either friends or acquaintances, compared with 44% in violence that came to the attention of the police [27]. Alcohol involvement in violence between 'good friends' was 55%, which was close to the mean for all episodes of violence. Risks relative to type of relationship could not be calculated because the time of being at risk was not known.

Alcohol dependence and friendship

In the study of the long-term effects of alcohol consumption it is accepted that inveterate drinking has negative consequences for relationships with friends, co-workers, family and other individuals in the drinker's social vicinity. Such consequences have been made into defining characteristics of alcohol dependence; scales of alcohol dependence include questions on difficulties with friends and family members as a result of drinking, such as: 'Were there major arguments in your family because of your drinking?' 'Did your drinking result in marital or family separation?' 'Did you lose friends because of your drinking?' Of course, such social consequences are only included in dependence scales if the scales discriminate between dependent and non-dependent individuals. These criteria are based on clinical studies that have shown that the consequences are common among alcoholics and heavy drinkers.

In assessing the impact of drinking on the nature and prevalence of different types of social relationship one would need to know, among other things, the extent to which friendships lost through problem drinking are replaced by other 'drinking friendships'. The importance and quality of relationships developed around heavy drinking are value-laden topics. The little that is known about group interaction among alcohol abusers indicates that solidarity may be at times strongly felt and expressed when alcohol is abundant and when the need arises to pool resources for buying a bottle. Relevant in this context is Rubington's [28] observation that some individuals in their misfortunes derive much solace from friendships formed in groups of alcohol abusers. Many former problem-drinkers affirm that giving up old friendships based on the heavy use of alcohol is a very difficult part of the change to sobriety, and meeting old drinking friends is a frequent cause of relapse [29].

Many groups of alcohol abusers experience much internal strife. Lenke [30] and other later Swedish researchers have found that a disproportionately high share of violent crimes occurs in groups of alcohol abusers. There are indications that violence in such friendship groups is underreported. They have mostly adversarial relationships with the police, and members are unlikely to report violent occurrences within the group. In addition, the police in some jurisdictions tend to disregard violence that occurs in groups of alcohol abusers, because it is so common and 'the victim one day may well be the assailant the next day'. The prevalence of stresses and strains in groups of alcohol abusers may differ between countries – beverage alcohol (or its substitutes) may cost less in some countries than in others, or living conditions (as determined by, for instance, climate) may be less stressful. Very little is known about this. Similarly, little is known about the effects of the more prevalent moderate to light drinking on friendships in modern societies. It is often argued in the anthropological literature that communal drinking as it is practised in small pre-industrialized societies has positive functions for the community and its individuals [31]. Ethnographic descriptions focus on central tendencies and shared belief systems, however, and functionalist interpretations by their very nature find positive consequences of persisting behaviour patterns, including alcohol consumption. It is difficult, nevertheless, to understand how communal drinking, including drinking with friends, would persist unless it had predominantly positive social consequences.

Engaging in unplanned sex; experiencing unwanted sexual advances

Categories of drinkers differ in their perceptions of the opportunity structure of drinking occasions. For an adolescent, a drinking event may be a way of gaining status in the group of friends, especially if it is combined with other risk-taking activities. It may also have other identity-shaping functions, such as advancing liberation from dependence on parents and parental control, and development towards adulthood.

Alcohol also plays various symbolic roles, related to the gender of a drinking group. The idea expressed in Ogden Nash's rhyme: 'Candy is dandy, but liquor is quicker', has probably guided plans for sexual encounters over the centuries.

Men more than women define mixed drinking-occasions as precursors of sexual relations [32]. To some men, alcohol and intoxication in women signal sexual availability [33]. The presence of a woman in a certain type of bar may have similar connotations [34]. Men accused of rape sometimes use these connotations as a defence. Alcohol also incapacitates the potential victim of sexual violence, and a sexually predatory male may see an intoxicated female acquaintance as an easy target.

Comparisons of different types of violent crime have shown that, while assailants usually attack strangers, rapists attack acquaintances [35]. Sexual assaults and 'date rapes' have raised concern in American universities, and several campuses have introduced prevention programmes. A study of one such intervention found that in three of every four such incidents off campus, and in seven of every eight on campus, the sexual assailants were known to the victims [36]. Alcohol intoxication is common among both offenders and victims of such assaults.

In the European School Survey Project on Alcohol and Other Drugs, countries differed widely (4–22%; females, 2–27%; males, 6–27%) in the proportions of students who felt that their drinking had caused them to 'engage in unwanted sexual experience' [15]. The likelihood of such occurrences did not seem to be strongly related to the general level of drinking among the youth of these countries and, consequently, little is known about the frequency with which unwanted sexual advances are an outcome of intoxication *per se*. Expectancies linked to alcohol seem to be important in this respect. There are probably cultural differences as to what is tolerated in connection with drinking, and definitions of drinking occasions as 'sexual time out' among youth may vary between countries or social classes, for instance. Also, behaviour related to alcohol may be determined more in some countries by its pharmacological properties and in others by its symbolism.

Cognitive impairment due to alcohol may cause individuals to misperceive or misinterpret the intent of others [37, 38]. It undoubtedly also increases the risk that women will inadvertently send interactional signals that in a sober context would be open invitations to a sexual encounter. In short, even among friends and acquaintances, men and women differ as to the symbolism and consequences of drinking. This is indicated by the date rapes and 'acquaintance rapes' that occur after drinking.

In the last 15 years much of the literature on sexual behaviour has dealt with the extent to which different groups of people, especially those perceived to be at high risk – drug abusers, male and female prostitutes, homeless youth, teenagers, practise safe sex. The most recent studies have found that, contrary to expectations, sexually active individuals practise safe sex no less often after drinking than when sober [39], which suggests that there may be a considerable element of rational planning in many sexual encounters under the influence of alcohol.

Whatever the cause or reason, sexual advances are probably more common

60 *Consequences of drinking to friends and the close social environment*

in connection with drinking than with sobriety. There are, undeniably, bars, so-called 'pick-up bars', where securing a sexual partner for the night is a major reason for frequenting it. In other drinking places one is likely to meet prostitutes. Such opportunity structures may in part explain some of the misconceptions in some societies regarding female drinking, even among groups of friends and acquaintances.

'Bracketing' or how to link two realities

Norwegian general-population surveys have measured the prevalence of being subjected to alcohol-related aggressive or annoying behaviour. Table 1 (from [40]) shows that bothersome behaviour by intoxicated people is not uncommon in this population and that the risk appears to be higher in urban centres. This table does not refer to the relationships in which these occurrences took place (or to the frequency of the occurrences). The occurrences in the street were probably due to strangers mainly.

Table 1 Proportion of the Norwegian and Oslo populations aged 15 years and over who had experienced different types of annoying or hazardous behaviour by intoxicated persons in the last 12 months

	All Norway	Oslo
Accosted or bothered in a public place	14%	24%
Accosted or bothered in a private setting	6%	8%
Received a physical injury	2%	3%
Had property destroyed	4%	6%
Verbally abused	16%	21%
Been afraid of intoxicated people in the street	14%	21%
Kept awake at night due to noise	19%	28%

The revellers who commit some of these nuisances are groups of friends who enjoy what to others are annoying experiences. The intoxicated in-group defines the situation differently from how the, mostly sober, outsiders define it.

Impulsive and spontaneous acts (and unpredictable and unexpected forms of interaction) characterize intoxicated behaviour. The unpredictable behaviour can be of both a negative and a positive nature. The rules that govern sober behaviour are broken – a characteristic sometimes referred to as 'time out'. Though 'time out' behaviour is identical with the disinhibiting, pharmacologically determined, effects of alcohol, the concept of 'time out' implies that behaviour after drinking is determined predominantly by social constructions surrounding alcohol. Alcohol-use events are viewed as socially defined occasions where people are allowed to behave in a way that would meet with disapproval if they were sober.

Social consequences of alcohol consumption depend in part on how society and significant others define the social consequentiality of drinking occasions and intoxicated behaviour. Mechanisms built into the cultural fabric act as buffers and transformers of the impact that intoxicated behaviour has on sober reality. The concept of 'time out' has been used widely to characterize a situation with specific norms for what is prescribed or accepted in alcohol-use situations [41]. A related concept is the cognitive activity of 'bracketing' part or all of what happens in an intoxicated state. These concepts imply that intoxication/alcohol-events are allowed to have separate rules from those that apply to sober behaviour.

The extent to which this type of bracketing occurs in modern societies has been little studied. Most of what is known is based on surveys of opinions concerning fictional crimes and not on observations of behaviour in everyday relationships. The findings regarding public views on the culpability of drunken offenders are somewhat inconclusive but do point to limitations on the extent to which bracketing may be used as a neutralizing tactic [42, 43]. The laws of many countries make no special provision for crimes committed under alcohol intoxication. In recent years there has been sustained public opposition to the legal bracketing of intoxication in regard to drunken driving and domestic violence. Legal practice, however, still leaves room for diversion of intoxicated offenders into treatment, and homicide is more likely in many countries to be treated as manslaughter than as murder when the perpetrator has been drinking (and, especially, if both victim and perpetrator have been drinking). There is no research on whether such a discrepancy between theory and practice exists also in the case of less serious infractions in social relationships.

A strict concept of 'time out' would imply that there is no carry-over from the alcohol occasion to the sober and consequential world. In modern society this assumption does not hold up, apart perhaps from small and homogeneous societies with communal drinking where an occasion is defined by tradition in a way that leaves little room for individual interpretations of its purpose and meaning. In the modern world, drinking occurs in so many different social contexts that it is impossible to generalize to all drinking events. Alcohol is often part of business luncheons and dinners. In some parts of the world, it is sometimes part of diplomatic negotiations, but treaties signed after very 'wet' negotiations cannot be annulled by appealing to 'time out'.

Social consequences of intoxicated behaviour in face-to-face relationships are more easily bracketed. Typical instances are described in Cavan's [44] classic study of San Francisco bars. She found, for instance, that personal identities presented in bars are inconsequential. No one seriously objects if someone representing himself to be an architect is later found to be working in a warehouse. Situational identities are one kind of reward sought in groups of drinkers. There is less cultural leeway for bracketing of long-term consequences of drinking.

CONCLUDING REMARKS

This chapter has stressed the reciprocal nature of drinking-related consequences in relationships between friends. An individual's drinking habits will affect those of his friends, and theirs in turn will affect his. Selection and deselection of associates and friends occurs mutually and is in part based on drinking habits and drinking behaviour. Unlike family, friends can be chosen and abandoned in this way. This fact may underlie major differences between the two social relationships with regard to the social consequences of drinking.

The social consequences of alcohol use in relation to different kinds of relationship may perhaps be represented as a J-shaped curve in perceived annoyances and problems. Annoyances caused by strangers are mainly transient, with few positive consequences; friends and acquaintances share in positive moods, camaraderie and revelry. With the closest relationships, immediate relatives, the negative aspects seem to predominate. This picture is simplistic, however; it does not fit all aspects of reality. A longitudinal study in a general population of drinkers might very well show that the time spent in positive alcohol-related situations would outweigh the negative in all social relationships. It is clear, however, that negative consequences of alcohol are strongly clustered to some close relationships. It is an open question, perhaps with no rationally based answer, whether sufficient alcohol-related positive moments could be found in many relationships to balance the alcohol-related fear and misery that a minority of relationships must endure.

The possibility of bracketing what occurs in drinking events, and the excuse value of intoxication, are used in society to decrease the damage done to personal relationships. The extent to which this is possible and successful is likely to differ between societies and over time in the same society, and also to be contingent on type of relationship.

To what extent can alcohol-related behaviour and the social consequences of alcohol be attributed to the chemical or pharmacological properties of alcohol, and to what extent are they attributable to social constructions associated with alcohol? The issue is far from settled, but there is an emerging consensus that there is a core of pharmacological effects that are relevant to this assessment. The effects that social beliefs regarding alcohol may have on alcohol-related behaviour have been widely researched and discussed during the last couple of decades. No firm conclusions can be drawn on the basis of this research except that many of the causal processes that link alcohol consumption with social outcomes are themselves social in nature.

The fact that social consequences may be based on social constructions makes them no less real – they are, however, less predictable. They are also more likely to change over time and to differ among cultures and subcultures. This, of course, sets limits to the types of generalization that can be made regarding social consequences. From the relevant literature it is easy to get the impression that the negative effects of alcohol predominate in human relationships.

Research interest, however, is not a good measure of the relative prevalence of positive and negative consequences. Negative effects cause more problems in society and are, therefore, studied in greater depth. They are also made the target of preventive efforts, which leads to further evaluative research, and to further 'biases' in the literature. This emphasis on the negative is not limited to research on alcohol. From the scientific literature on sexual behaviour, for instance, one may easily get the impression that human love-making is a problem area, dominated by unwanted sexual advances, rape and sexually transmitted diseases.

Value judgments are implicit in much of the assessment made about the social consequences of alcohol. In some cases the moral attitude chosen may seem self-evident, as in the case of violent behaviour, unwanted sexual advances linked to drinking, and deleterious consequences to children and to family life. When we try to assess the positive effects that alcohol undeniably has, our moral stance is probably not so obvious.

Moderate drinking may have positive effects on friendships and other relationships, as it has for physical (and possibly mental) health. As with health consequences, the main challenge is to ensure that the most drinkers stay within the limits that safeguard healthy human relationships.

REFERENCES

1. Aas, H. and Klepp, K.I. (1992) Adolescents' alcohol use related to perceived norms. *Scandinavian Journal of Psychology* **33**(4), 315–325.
2. Barnes, G.M. and Farrell, M.P. (1992) Parental support and control as predictors of adolescent drinking, delinquency, and related problem behaviors. *Journal of Marriage and the Family* **54**(4), 763–776.
3. Basten, C.J. and Kavanagh, D.J. (1996) Alcohol consumption by undergraduate students. *Substance Use and Misuse* **31**(10), 1379–1399.
4. Mason, C.A. et al. (1994) Adolescent problem behavior - the effect of peers and the moderating role of father absence and the mother-child relationship. *American Journal of Community Psychology* **22**(6), 723–743.
5. Ndom, R.J.E. and Adelekan, M.L. (1996) Psychosocial correlates of substance use among undergraduates in Ilorin University, Nigeria. *East African Medical Journal* **73**(8), 541–547.
6. Clapper, R.L. et al. (1995) Adolescent problem behaviors as predictors of adult alcohol diagnoses. *International Journal of the Addictions* **30**(5), 507–523.
7. Schulenberg, J. et al. (1999) On peer influence to get drunk: A panel study of young adolescents. *Merrill-Palmer Quarterly Journal of Developmental Psychology* **45**(1), 108–142.
8. Reed, M.D. and Rountree, P.W. (1997) Peer pressure and adolescent substance use. *Journal of Quantitative Criminology* **13**(2), 143–180.
9. Skog, O.-J. (1980) Social interaction and the distribution of alcohol consumption. *Journal of Drug Issues* **10**(1), 71–92.
10. Dishion, T.J. et al. (1999) Middle childhood antecedents to progressions in male adolescent substance use: an ecological analysis of risk and protection. *Journal of Adolescent Research* **14**(2), 175–205.

11. Zhang, L.N. et al. (1997) The impact of age of onset of substance use on delinquency. *Journal of Research in Crime and Delinquency* **34**(2), 253–268.
12. Bogenschneider, K. et al. (1998) 'Other teens drink, but not my kid': Does parental awareness of adolescent alcohol use protect adolescents from risky consequences? *Journal of Marriage and the Family* **60**(2), 356–373.
13. Lindström, P. (1996) Family interaction, neighbourhood context and deviant behaviour: A research note. *Studies on Crime and Crime Prevention* **5**(1), 1–11.
14. Skretting, A. (1999) *Bruk av rusmidler ved utgangen av ungdomsskolen* [Use of intoxicants at the end of junior public school], National Institute for Alcohol and Drug Research, Oslo.
15. Hibell, B. et al. (1996) *The ESPAD Report. Alcohol and Drug Use among Students in 26 European Countries*, The Swedish Council for Information on Alcohol and Other Drugs and The Pompidou Group at the Council of Europe, Stockholm.
16. Pope, S.K. et al. (1994) Gender differences in rural adolescent drinking patterns. *Journal of Adolescent Health* **15**(5), 359–365.
17. Corcoran, K.M. and Michels, J.L. (1998) A prototype analysis of psychological situations through the lens of alcohol expectancies and gender. *Addictive Behaviors* **23**(5), 685–691.
18. Pernanen, K. (1976) Alcohol and crimes of violence, in *The Biology of Alcoholism: Vol 4 Social Aspects of Alcoholism* (eds B. Kissin and H. Begleiter), Plenum Press, New York, pp. 351–444.
19. Pernanen, K. (1993) Alcohol-related violence: Conceptual models and methodological issues, in *Alcohol and Interpersonal Violence: Fostering Multidisciplinary Perspectives* (ed. S. Martin), US Department of Health and Human Services, National Institute of Alcohol Abuse and Alcoholism, Washington DC (Research Monograph 24).
20. Taylor, S. and Leonard, K.E. (1983) Alcohol and human physical aggression, in *Aggression: Theoretical and Empirical Reviews* (eds. R.G. Geen and E.I. Donnerstein), Academic Press, New York, (2, Issues in research).
21. Smith, M.J. et al. (1993) Reasons for drinking – their relationship to psychosocial variables and alcohol consumption. *International Journal of the Addictions* **28**(9), 881–908.
22. Webb, J.A. et al. (1999) Intentions to use alcohol among fifth and sixth graders: The roles of social and stress/coping motives. *American Journal of Orthopsychiatry* **69**(4), 541–547.
23. Duka, T. et al. (1998) Alcohol choice and outcome expectancies in social drinkers. *Behavioural Pharmacology* **9**(7), 643–653.
24. Kilbey, M.M. et al. (1998) Predicting the emergence and persistence of alcohol dependence in young adults: the role of expectancy and other risk factors. *Experimental and Clinical Psychopharmacology* **6**(2), 149–156.
25. Yokoyama, K. et al. (1999) Reasons for drinking in relation to problem drinking behavior in a sample of Japanese high school students. *International Journal of Behavioral Medicine* **6**(2), 135–149.
26. Wright, S.W. and Slovis, C.M. (1996) Drinking on campus – Undergraduate intoxication requiring emergency care. *Archives of Pediatrics and Adolescent Medicine* **150**(7), 699–702.
27. Pernanen, K. (1991) *Alcohol in Human Violence*, Guilford Press, New York.
28. Rubington, E. (1977) 'Failure' as a heavy drinker: the case of the chronic-drunkenness offender on Skid Row, in *Society, Culture, and Drinking Patterns* (eds D.J. Pittman and C.R. Snyder), Southern Illinois University Press, Carbondale, Edwardsville, pp. 146–187.
29. Newlove, D. (1988) *Those Drinking Days; Myself and Other Writers*, McGraw-Hill, New York.

30. Lenke, L. (1974) *Våldsbrottsligheten i Stockholm* [Crimes of violence in Stockholm], University of Stockholm: Institute of Criminology, Stockholm.
31. Heath, D.B. (1958) Drinking patterns of the Bolivian Camba. *Quarterly Journal of Studies on Alcohol* **19**, 491–508.
32. Mongeau, P.A. and Johnson, K.L. (1995) Predicting cross-sex first-date sexual expectations and involvement: Contextual and individual difference factors. *Personal Relationships* **2**(4), 301–312.
33. George, W.H. *et al.* (1997) Postdrinking sexual inferences: evidence for linear rather than curvilinear dosage effects. *Journal of Applied Social Psychology* **27**(7), 629–648.
34. Parks, K.A. and Miller, B.A. (1997) Bar victimization of women. *Psychology of Women Quarterly* **21**(4), 509–525.
35. Gudjonsson, G.H. and Sigurdsson, J.F. (2000) Differences and similarities between violent offenders and sex offenders. *Child Abuse and Neglect* **24**(3), 363–372.
36. Meilman, P.W. and Haygood Jackson, D. (1996) Data on sexual assault from the first 2 years of a comprehensive campus prevention program. *Journal of American College Health* **44**(4), 157–165.
37. Abbey, A. *et al.* (1998) Sexual assault perpetration by college men: the role of alcohol, misperception of sexual intent, and sexual beliefs and experiences. *Journal of Social and Clinical Psychology* **17**(2), 167–195.
38. Gillen, K. and Muncer, S.J. (1995) Sex differences in the perceived causal structure of date rape – a preliminary report. *Aggressive Behaviour* **21**(2), 101–112.
39. Graves, K.L. and Leigh, B.C. (1995) The relationship of substance use to sexual activity among young adults in the United States. *Familiy Planning Perspectives* **27**(1), 18–27.
40. Amundsen, A. *et al.* (1995) *Alkohol og narkotika i Oslo* [Alcohol and Drugs in Oslo], National Institute for Alcohol and Drug Research, Oslo.
41. MacAndrew, C. and Edgerton, R.B. (1969) *Drunken Comportment*, Aldine, Chicago.
42. Schuller, R.A. and Wall, A.M. (1998) The effects of defendant and complainant intoxication on mock jurors' judgments of sexual assault. *Psychology of Women Quarterly* **22**(4), 555–573.
43. Wild, T.C. *et al.* (1998) Blame and punishment for intoxicated aggression: when is the perpetrator culpable? *Addiction* **93**(5), 677–687.
44. Cavan, S. (1966) *Liquor License: An Ethnography of Bar Behaviour*, Aldine, Chicago.

Chapter five

The impact of alcohol consumption on work and education

J. Rehm and I. Rossow

This chapter is primarily about the consequences of drinking that affect participation and productivity in work and participation and achievement in education. Work-related accidents and injuries are discussed in Chapter 7.

WORK

Alcohol surveys in general include questions on work problems related to alcohol, usually as part of a series of questions on different kinds of experienced alcohol-related harm [1]. Of these, at least in North America, alcohol-related harm to health is the most often indicated [1, 2], followed by financial problems. Work problems related to alcohol use are less common in terms of prevalence, but still result in public-health relevant absolute numbers in North America and Europe. In Canada, for example, 4.6% of male and 1.8% of female current drinkers had experienced alcohol-related problems with work, studies or employment during the twelve months preceding a recent survey [1]; and 11.4% of the male and 4.7% of the female current drinkers had experienced such problems at least once in their lives. Finally, 22.0% of male former drinkers and 9.6% of female former drinkers had lifetime alcohol-related work problems, which may have been a reason for many of them to quit drinking. Although this approach may have methodological flaws [3] (see also Chapter 3 for a detailed discussion of this), these numbers indicate that alcohol-related work problems

Harald Klingemann and Gerhard Gmel (eds.), Mapping the Social Consequences of Alcohol Consumption, 67–77.
© 2001 *Kluwer Academic Publishers. Printed in Great Britain.*

are highly prevalent. This is confirmed by the extremely high social costs of alcohol-related productivity losses and other workplace-related problems in most established market economies [4, 5, 6; also Table 9, for an overview of studies on economic costs of alcohol in the workplace].

The pervasiveness of alcohol-related work problems is not surprising, since in many market economies many workers drink on the job. Estimates from studies in different companies in the United States range from 2% to 15%, and a representative national Canadian survey in 1991 found that 22% of the workforce drank on the job [6, Table 2].

While these general population surveys referred to work as such, irrespective of type of problem, other research has specified the following types of alcohol-related problem [6, 7]:

- workplace accidents resulting in death or injury (covered in Chapter 8)
- absenteeism (including tardiness and leaving work early) due to illness, or disciplinary suspension, resulting in loss of productivity
- turnover due to premature death, disciplinary problems or low productivity from the use of alcohol
- inappropriate behaviour (such as behaviour resulting in disciplinary procedures)
- theft and other crime
- poor co-worker relations and low company morale.

This chapter first considers research in relation to two broad categories of those types of problem: alcohol consumption and absenteeism, and alcohol consumption and other work problems. A discussion of moderating and modifying variables follows, and the section on work closes with a discussion of drinking patterns most related to workplace problems.

First, however, in what way does absenteeism constitute social harm? According to the definition of social consequences in Chapter 1, one of the characteristics of social consequences is the influence or effect of one person's actions or behaviour on others. Absenteeism directly affects the employer, and possibly also co-workers and customers; indirectly, through its social costs, it affects others [8]. Thus, absenteeism constitutes social harm in the sense used in this volume.

ALCOHOL AND ABSENTEEISM

Sickness absence entails a substantial cost to employers and social security systems. It is mostly attributable to chronic diseases, often musculoskeletal or respiratory, and to mental disorders, but empirical studies of sickness absence have shown a considerable effect of alcohol use and abuse. Thus, since the early work of Stevenson [9], there is ample evidence that alcohol dependents and problem drinkers have higher rates of sickness absence than other employees, and that pay received by employees while on sick-leave in this group amounts to much more than in other groups of employees [10–29].

This evidence comes from different types and methods of study. In some of the earlier studies, recovered problem drinkers were asked about their absenteeism during their periods of problem drinking [11, 12]. Most of the studies combined self-reported estimations of alcohol consumption with either self-reported or objective data on sick days of the individuals concerned. Some studies, however, also asked about tardiness or absence from work of other employees [19]. One study used a quasi-experimental design to assess a drop in absenteeism and in amount of sickness benefit paid after alcohol testing had been established [16]. All of those studies found a higher rate of absenteeism among problem drinkers (often defined in categories of volume) or alcohol dependents than among low risk drinkers, though some studies found such results only in males [20, 22].

The numbers of absent days attributable to alcohol consumption vary considerably by industry, time and region. A study on alcohol-related sickness-absence in Norway has shown that it represents only around 1.5% to 2% of the total amount of sickness absence. Yet, alcohol-related absenteeism seems to constitute a significant proportion of the short-term sickness absence in Norway with a liberal sick-pay scheme. There, 15–20% of all absenteeism of less than four days, and perhaps as much as 40% of all sickness absences of one day, was estimated to be alcohol-related [28].

A number of studies have estimated the costs of alcohol-related sickness-absence. Hocking and co-workers [23] in Australia, for instance, estimated the cost of alcohol-related absenteeism to be approximately A$ 90 per employee per year. Marmot and colleagues [22] found that in Great Britain absenteeism related to alcohol cost an annual total of £779 million. These estimates were based largely on data on heavy drinkers, as the evidence relating to moderate drinkers was less clear. According to the theoretical model of the preventive paradox [30], however, moderate drinkers who occasionally drink heavily would account for most such absenteeism. This hypothesis is supported by two population-based studies from New Zealand [15, 25], which assessed alcohol-related absenteeism and its costs in relation to self-reported alcohol consumption. Casswell and co-workers [15] found that 18% of those who reported alcohol-related sickness-absence came from the 4.5% of the respondents considered to be heavy drinkers. In the later study of Jones and co-workers [25], 42% of the alcohol-related sickness-absence days and 46% of the cost were found to be attributable to the upper 10% of the drinkers. A Nordic comparative study [29] found that between a fourth and a third of alcohol-related absenteeism could be attributed to the heavy drinkers. Whether the preventive paradox is valid for sickness absence related to alcohol, however, may dependent on a number of factors, such as drinking culture, labour-market conditions and sick-pay schemes.

ALCOHOL-RELATED WORK PROBLEMS OTHER THAN ABSENTEEISM

A number of studies have demonstrated an association between heavy drinking or alcohol abuse and unemployment [31–36]. Here, a causal association may go in either direction: heavy drinking may lead to unemployment, as suggested by Mustonen et al. [32] and Mullahy and Sindelar [31]; but loss of work may cause an increase in drinking, which may become heavy drinking, as indicated by Claussen [36], Gallant [33] and Dooley and Prause [37].

Kandel and Yamaguchi [38] reported that, in New England, young-adult employees who drank daily held their jobs for shorter periods than others. Blum et al. [39] and Mangione et al. [40] found that work performance was related to volume and pattern of drinking (see below). In the Blum et al. study, lower performance, lack of self-direction and problems in personal relations were found to be related to heavy drinking. The already mentioned Alberta Alcohol and Drug Abuse Commission (AADAC) survey of workers, employers and union officials in Alberta, Canada, found that 22% of the workers were aware of one or more incidents related to the use of alcohol or drugs, ranging from slight physical impairment to criminal behaviour or extended absence due to substance abuse.

INTERACTION OF ALCOHOL CONSUMPTION WITH OTHER FACTORS

The contribution of alcohol to work problems depends also on other factors. Grunberg and colleagues [41] found, for example, a strong effect of reasons for drinking and stress. Higher prevalence of drinking-related work problems was associated with higher levels of job stress only for those who gave escapist reasons for drinking. For others, more stress led to less drinking and fewer alcohol-related problems.

In general, according to the theoretical model of Ames and Jane [42] the factors influencing the relation between alcohol and work problems may be summarized under the following broad headings:

- normative regulation of drinking
- drinking subcultures
- quality and organization of work
- other workplace factors.

Macdonald, Wells and Wild [43] found some empirical support for this approach.

DRINKING PATTERNS ASSOCIATED WITH WORKPLACE PROBLEMS

While this chapter cannot go into detail on all the complex interactions between characteristics of work, drinking and related problems, we will try to describe which style of drinking *ceteris paribus* was associated with work problems. Recent research has shown that heavy-drinking occasions and drinking on the job are more predictive of workplace problems than average volume. Mangione and colleagues [40] found, for instance, that in a multivariate regression that controlled for a number of demographic variables, job characteristics and life-situations, average daily volume was no longer significantly associated with the number of times respondents experienced problems related with poorer work-performance during the previous year. By contrast, measures of alcohol dependence (CAGE), frequency of getting drunk, and drinking during any of six workday situations were significant determinants of work-performance. Ames, Grube and Moore [27], showing that, in bivariate analyses, only overall drinking and heavy drinking outside the workplace predicted workplace problems, have reported very similar findings. In multivariate analyses, the influence of these factors was no longer found significant, but workplace drinking and coming to work with a hangover predicted work-related problems even when usual patterns, heavy drinking, job characteristics and sociodemographic background variables were controlled for. Finally, Midanik and colleagues [44] found that, controlling for volume, respondents who had reported heavy drinking occasions during the previous year (as defined by 5 or more drinks per occasion) were at significantly higher risk of work problems.

Taken together, these results constitute convincing evidence of a strong determinant effect of heavy drinking occasions and workplace drinking on the occurrence of alcohol-related work problems. Efforts to prevent such problems should be directed at those determinants – for example, by the adoption and implementation of policies limiting or prohibiting drinking on the job or by providing work-site information and education designed to help all employees understand the relationship between drinking behaviour and work performance [40].

EDUCATION

Pupils and students in educational systems are generally young, and thus the consequences of alcohol consumption in the form of school dropout, poor scholastic performance and educational underachievement are primarily short-term effects of drinking rather than long-term effects of prolonged heavy drinking. Obviously, also, parental drinking affects children's scholastic performance. This may be in part a long-term effect of maternal drinking during pregnancy: young schoolchildren who were exposed prenatally to alcohol may manifest attention deficits and behavioural problems [45]. Also, Olson and co-workers [46] found a significant dose-response relationship between prenatal exposure to alcohol and attentional difficulties, classroom hyperactivity, difficulty in information processing, and academic difficulties at the age of 11, all typical long-lasting effects of maternal drinking during pregnancy on scholastic performance. Beyond pregnancy, parental drinking affects the child in other ways. In retrospective interviews with children, for instance, Robins et al. [47] found that having an alcoholic father was associated with truancy and dropout. Later studies have demonstrated that poor performance at school is related to poor parental attachment and lack of parental care [48], which may, therefore, be one kind of mediator of the observed relationship between parental drinking and a child's scholastic performance.

Here, however, we are concerned with the association between drinking on the part of the student or schoolchild and various social problems related to education. Truancy and dropout are observed more often among heavy drinkers or the frequently intoxicated [48–51]. Truancy would be expected to follow from hangovers and sleepiness after episodes of heavy drinking. Wichstrøm [48], however, found no empirical support for this; he found, rather, a bi-directional relationship between alcoholic intoxication and playing truant – 'wanting to do something else', rather than tiredness or sleepiness, was a strong motive for truancy. A bivariate association between intoxication and dropout observed in Wichstrøm's study [48] was in part spurious, attributable to lack of parental care, but also mediated in two ways:

- intoxication increasing the risk of truancy and thereby school dropout
- intoxication leading to differential association with peers with high involvment in problem behaviour, which in turn favours school dropout.

In line with these results, the findings of Costa et al. [51] indicated a clustering of problem drinking, peer models for substance use, and poor scholastic performance. Kasen et al. [52] also noted that poor performance at school, truancy and dropout were associated with having deviant friends in adolescence. Moreover, Wood et al. [53] found that the association between problem drinking and academic problems in college was attributable mostly to pre-existing problem-behaviour.

Students may employ self-handicapping 'strategies' to account for poor scholastic performance: they may try to portray their poor performance at school as due to circumstances that prevent them from studying rather than to lack of ability [54]. Their choice of deviant friends may be viewed in this perspective. From a series of surveys of Norwegian youth, Rossow and Skretting (forthcoming) found that fewer than 1% of a sample of more than 17 000 students aged 15–20 years had experienced any kind of school problem that they attributed to their own drinking during the previous 6 months. This proportion increased with total alcohol consumption and frequency of intoxication, and among the heaviest drinkers (reporting drinking to intoxication at least once a week) 10% reported school problems due to their own drinking in the previous 6 months. It is noteworthy that poor performance at school, truancy and dropout predict later heavy drinking and alcohol problems [55, 56]. This may indicate a spiral of increasing deviance or maladjustment in the association between drinking behaviour, on the one hand, and, on the other, participation and performance in education and the labour market.

One of the social aspects of drinking among students is pressure to drink. A number of studies have demonstrated a strong association between students' self-reported drinking habits and what they perceive as those of their adolescent and young-adult peers [57–60]. Adolescents form and maintain friendships from the experience of common drinking behaviour and lifestyle, owing primarily to the social nature of drinking and to the occurrence of adolescent drinking mostly at parties or social events where proximity and shared experience conduce to forming friendships. The alcohol expectancies of adolescents are primarily along a social dimension, which is also the dimension of alcohol expectancy most strongly associated with drinking behaviour [60–62]. Thus, expectations of enhanced social relations seem to be the strongest motive for young people's drinking, and these expectations also appear to be reinforced with increased drinking. Yet, several studies have found that young people's perceptions of the drinking behaviour of friends are exaggerated [60], and thus correspondingly the perceived pressure to drink. In recent years explanations for such a fictitious norm pressure to drink have been debated. Pedersen [63] suggested two explanations:

- there may be a 'false consensus' in the sense that adolescents exaggerate to themselves the extent to which their own norms and behaviour are shared by their reference groups;

- 'asymmetric ties': individuals with the more deviant behaviour and norms have larger social networks and thus are more often found in young people's reference groups.

Mäkelä [64], however, has suggested that, by exaggerating the drinking behaviour of significant others, the adolescent's own cognitive dissonance is reduced, and this would be particularly the case in restrictive communities and among those with negative attitudes to alcohol. As drinking is very much a social form of behaviour that takes place in the company of other people, the association between drinking and social skills or social competence becomes an issue. A few studies have touched upon this, although their findings are not consistent. Leifman and co-workers [65] found that young light and moderate drinkers had a better developed social network than abstainers, and Pape and Hammer [66] as well as Holtung and Rossow [67] have reported similar findings. Hover and Gaffney [68] found, however, that adolescent problem drinkers were more often than other drinkers incompetent in social skills, and that non-drinkers were most often in the highly competent range.

REFERENCES

1. Rehm, J. et al. (1999) A reliability and validity analysis of an alcohol-related harm scale for surveys. *Journal of Studies on Alcohol* **60**(2), 203–208.
2. Single, E. et al. (1995) Nineteen ninety three (1993) General Social Survey I: alcohol use in Canada. *Canadian Journal of Public Health* **86**, 397–401.
3. Rehm, J. and Gmel, G. (1999) Patterns of alcohol consumption and social consequences. Results from an 8-year follow-up study in Switzerland. *Addiction* **94**(6), 899–912.
4. Single, E. et al. (1998) The economic costs of alcohol, tobacco and illicit drugs in Canada, 1992. *Addiction* **93**(7), 991–1006.
5. Xie, X. et al. (1998) The economic costs of alcohol abuse in Ontario. *Pharmacological Research* **37**, 241–249.
6. Single, E. (1998) *Substance Abuse and the Workplace in Canada*, Canadian Centre on Substance Abuse, Ottawa, (Report prepared for Health Canada on behalf of the Canadian Centre on Substance Abuse).
7. International Labour Office (ILO). (1998) *Substance Abuse and the Workplace: Current State of Research and Future Needs*, International Labour Office, Geneva.
8. Single, E. et al. (1996) *The Costs of Substance Abuse in Canada*, Canadian Centre on Substance Abuse, Ottawa.
9. Stevenson, R. (1942) Absenteeism in an industrial plant due to alcoholism. *Quarterly Journal of Studies on Alcohol* **2**, 661–668.
10. Lingren, G. (1957) Alkohol och arbete. [Alcohol and work] *Svenska Lakatidn* **54**, 3613–3620.
11. Maxwell, M. (1960) Early identification of problem drinkers in industry. *Quarterly Journal of Studies on Alcohol* **21**, 655–678.
12. Trice, H. (1965) Alcoholic employees – a comparison of psychotic, neurotic and 'normal' personnel. *Journal of Occupational Medicine* **7**, 94–99.
13. Schlosser, D. and McBride, J.W. (1984) *Estimating the Prevalence of Alcohol and Other Drug Related Problems in Industry*, New South Wales Drug and Alcohol Authority Research, Sydney, (Grant Report Series No. B84/3).
14. Beaumont, P.B. and Hyman, J. (1987) The work performance indicators of problem drinking: some British evidence. *Journal of Occupational Behavior* **8**, 55–62.
15. Casswell, S. et al. (1988) Estimating alcohol-related absenteeism in New Zealand. *British Journal of Addiction* **83**(6), 677–682.
16. Taggart, R.W. (1989) Results of the drug testing program at Southern Pacific Railroad, in *Drugs in the Workplace: Research and Evaluation Data* (eds S.W. Gust and J.M. Walsh), National Institute on Drug Abuse, Rockville, (NIDA Research Monograph 91).
17. Pell, S. and D'Alonzo, C.A. (1970) Sickness absenteeism of alcoholics. *Journal of Occupational Medicine* **12**, 198–210.
18. Rosenbaum, A. et al. (1992) *Prevalance of Substance Use and Its Association With Performance Among Municipal Workers in a Southwestern City*, Institute of Behavioral Research, Forth Worth.
19. Alberta Alcohol and Drug Abuse Commission (AADAC). (1992) *Substance Use and the Alberta Workplace: The Prevalence and Impacts of Alcohol and Other Drugs*, Alcohol and Drug Abuse Commission, Edmonton, Alberta (Final Report).
20. Joeman, L.M. (1992) *Alcohol Consumption and Sickness Absence. An Analysis of 1984 General Household Survey Data*, Department of Employment, London.
21. Kleinsorge, G. (1993) *Germany: Drug and Alcohol Testing in the Workplace*, Report of the Interregional Tripartite Experts Meeting, Oslo.

22. Marmot, M.G. et al. (1993) Alcohol consumption and sickness absence from the Whitehall II study. *Addiction* **88**, 369–382.
23. Hocking, B. et al. (1994) Cost to industry of illnesses related to alcohol and smoking. A study of Telecom Australian employees. *The Medical Journal of Australia* **161**, 407–412.
24. Webb, G.R. et al. (1994) Relationships between high-risk and problem drinking and the occurrence of work injuries and related absences. *Journal of Studies on Alcohol* **55**, 434–446.
25. Jones, S. et al. (1995) The economic costs of alcohol related absenteeism and reduced productivity among the working population of New Zealand. *Addiction* **90**, 1455–1461.
26. Poikolainen, K. (1996) Alcohol and overall health outcomes, *Annals of Medicine* **28**, 381–384.
27. Ames, G.M. et al. (1997) The relationship of drinking and hangovers to workplace problems: an empirical study. *Journal of Studies on Alcohol* **58**(1), 37–47.
28. Grimsmo, A. and Rossow, I. (1997) Alcohol og sykefravær [Alcohol and Sickness Absence], National Institute for Alcohol and Drug Research, Oslo (Report series).
29. Rossow, I. et al. (1999) *The Wrath of Grapes. Alcohol Related Sickness Absence in the Nordic Countries*, Paper presented at the 25th Annual Alcohol Epidemiology Symposium of the Kettil Bruun Society, Montreal.
30. Kreitman, N. (1986) Alcohol consumption and the preventive paradox, *British Journal of Addiction* **81**, 353–363.
31. Mullahy, J. and Sindelar, J. (1996) Employment, unemployment and problem drinking. *Journal of Health Economics* **15**, 409–434.
32. Mustonen, H. et al. (1994) Drinking habits among the employed and unemployed. *Nordisk Alkoholtidskrift [Nordic Alcohol Studies]* English Supplement **11**, 21–34.
33. Gallant, D.M. (1993) Unemployment and ethanol consumption. *Alcoholism: Clinical and Experimental Research* **17**, 722.
34. Luoto, R. et al. (1998) Unemployment, sociodemographic background and consumption of alcohol before and during the economic recession of the 1990s in Finland. *International Journal of Epidemiology* **27**, 623–629.
35. Montgomery, S.M. et al. (1998) Unemployment, cigarette smoking, alcohol consumption and body weight in young British men. *European Journal of Public Health* **8**, 21–27.
36. Claussen, B. (1999) Alcohol disorders and re-employment in a 5-year follow-up of long-term unemployed. *Addiction* **94**, 133–138.
37. Dooley, D. and Prause, J. (1998) Underemployment and alcohol misuse in the National Longitudinal Survey of Youth. *Journal of Studies on Alcohol* **59**, 669–680.
38. Kandel, D. and Yamaguchi, K. (1987) Job mobility and drug use: an event history analysis. *American Journal of Sociology* **92**, 836–878.
39. Blum, T.C. et al. (1993) Alcohol consumption and work performance. *Journal of Studies on Alcohol* **54**, 61–70.
40. Mangione, T.W. et al. (1999) Employee drinking practices and work performance. *Journal of Studies on Alcohol* **60**, 261–270.
41. Grunberg, L. et al. (1999) Work stress and self-reported alcohol use: the moderating role of escapist reasons for drinking. *Journal of Occupational Health Psychology* **4**, 29–36.
42. Ames, G. (1993) Research and strategies for the primary prevention of workplace alcohol problems. *Alcohol Health and Research World* **17**, 19–27.
43. Macdonald, S. et al. (1999) Occupational risk factors associated with alcohol and drug problems. *American Journal of Drug and Alcohol Abuse* **25**, 351–369.
44. Midanik, L.T. et al. (1996) Risk functions for alcohol-related problems in a 1988 US national sample. *Addiction* **91**, 1427–1437.

45. Brown, R.T. et al. (1991) Effects of prenatal alcohol exposure at school age: II. Attention and behavior. *Neurotoxicology and Teratology* 13, 369–376.
46. Olson, H.C. et al. (1992) Prenatal exposure to alcohol and school problems in late childhood: a longitudinal prospective study. *Development and Pschopathology* 4, 341–359.
47. Robins, L.N. et al. (1978) Father's alcoholism and children's outcomes, in *Currents in Alcoholism: Psychiatric, Psychological, Social, and Epidemiological Studies* (ed. F.A. Seixas), Grune and Stratton, New York, pp. 313–372 (Volume IV).
48. Wichstrøm, L. (1998) Alcohol intoxication and school dropout. *Drug and Alcohol Review* 17, 413–421.
49. Morgan, M. et al. (1999) ESPAD Study: implications for prevention. *Drugs: Education, Prevention and Policy* 6, 243–256.
50. O'Malley, P.M. et al. (1998) Alcohol use among adolescents. *Alcohol Health and Research World* 22, 85–93.
51. Costa, F.M. et al. (1999) Transition into adolescent problem drinking: the role of psychosocial risk and protective factors. *Journal of Studies on Alcohol* 60, 480–490.
52. Kasen, S. et al. (1998) Adolescent school experiences and dropout, adolescent pregnancy, and young adult deviant behavior. *Journal of Adolescent Health* 13, 49–72.
53. Wood, P.K. et al. (1997) Predicting academic problems in college from freshman alcohol involvement. *Journal of Studies on Alcohol* 58, 200–210.
54. Midgley, C. and Urdan, T. (1995) Predictors of school students use of self-handicapping strategies. *Journal of Early Adolescence* 15, 389–411.
55. Karlsson, G. and Romelsjö, A. (1997) Longitudinal study of social, psychological and behavioural factors associated with drunken driving and public drunkenness. *Addiction* 92, 447–457.
56. Crum, R.M. et al. (1998) The association of educational achievement and school dropout with risk of alcoholism: a twenty-five-year prospective study of inner-city children. *Journal of Studies on Alcohol* 59, 318–326.
57. Biddle, B.J. et al. (1980) Parental and peer influence on adolescents. *Social Forces* 58, 1057–1079.
58. Norman, R.M.G. (1986) *The Nature and Correlates of Health Behavior*, Health Promotion Directorate, Ottawa, Canada.
59. Lau, R.R. et al. (1990) Development and change of young adults' preventive health beliefs and behavior: influence from parents and peers. *Journal of Health and Social Behavior* 31, 240–259.
60. Aas, H.N. (1995) *Adolescents' Alcohol Consumption and Alcohol Expectancies*, Dissertation, National Institute for Alcohol and Drug Research, Oslo.
61. Leigh, B.C. (1990) Alcohol and expectancies and reasons for drinking: comments from a study of sexuality. *Psychology of Addictive Behaviors* 4, 91–96.
62. Leigh, B.C. and Stacy, A.W. (1994) Self-generated alcohol outcome expectancies in four samples of drinkers. *Addiction Research* 1, 335–348.
63. Pedersen, W. (1993) The majority fallacy reconsidered. *Acta Sociologica* 36, 343–355.
64. Mäkelä, K. (1997) Drinking, the majority fallacy, cognitive dissonance and social pressure. *Addiction* 92, 729–736.
65. Leifman, H. et al. (1995) Abstinence in late adolescence: antecedents to and covariates of a sober lifestyle and its consequences. *Social Science and Medicine* 41, 113–121.
66. Pape, H. and Hammer, T. (1996) Sober adolescence – predictor of psychosocial maladjustment in young adulthood? *Scandinavian Journal of Psychology* 37, 362–377.

67. Holtung, A. and Rossow, I. (2000) Abstinence in young adulthood: psychosocial characteristics and impact of parental drinking habits. *Nordic Studies on Alcohol and Drugs* **17**, 57–67.
68. Hover, S. and Gaffney, L.R. (1991) Relationship between social skills and adolescent drinking. *Alcohol and Alcoholism* **26**, 207–214.

Chapter six

Problem drinking and relatives

E. Maffli

INTRODUCTION

Attention to the negative effects of excessive alcohol is currently accorded largely to the drinker and very much less to the drinker's immediate relatives. Historically, however, images of distressed families were what to a large extent contributed to the founding of the temperance movements and the attempts at treatment that occurred in the first half of the 20th century [1]. The progressive introduction of state welfare systems in a number of countries has perhaps helped to modify the more extreme aspects of the experiences of the immediate relatives of heavy drinkers, but what we know at present about their situation still gives cause for concern.

Numerous epidemiological studies [2–5] have highlighted the protective effects against the occurrence of alcohol-related problems of living as a couple, being married and raising children. Nevertheless, a large proportion of problem drinkers do live as a member of a couple or have close family ties. It may be assumed that other drinkers living alone had such ties in the past but that they were broken because of alcohol-related problems [6]. Clearly, such problems affect intimately many people other than the actual drinkers. According to conservative estimates, for each person who abuses alcohol, at least one other suffers directly as a consequence [7]. Other estimates, relating more to the number of persons affected more or less directly, are much higher [8].

The harm suffered by significant others (principally the partner or the children) varies. Sometimes it appears serious and irreversible – impairment of fetal development, for example, or neglect of very young children – but it may also be temporary and have no long-term consequences (e.g. shortage of money, relationship problems). Very broadly, and excluding the harm due to direct exposure (such as fetal alcohol syndrome), the consequences to those close to problem drinkers are of three types: (1) abusive or other forms of unacceptable behaviour towards immediate relatives on the part of the drinker while under the influence of alcohol – such behaviour may sometimes be extremely traumatic (e.g. sexual abuse, physical violence, neglect of duties of care); (2) economic and social, which have a less direct effect but which may place the household in a precarious position and socially isolate its members (owing among other reasons to the want of money spent on drink, or loss of income because of difficulties at work or loss of employment); and (3) relational, which are more complex to assess and may have as one of their obvious (and, sometimes paradoxically, healthy) outcomes the split or break-up of the family. These different types are likely to overlap or to interact with one another, with consequent considerable distress in many cases.

This preliminary review would be incomplete without mention of the possible 'contamination' effect of the drinker's behaviour on immediate relatives. The behavioural model presented by the drinker, and the suffering or degradation endured by immediate relatives, contribute to a predisposition to the use of alcohol among family members – sometimes several years later – thus creating a vicious circle which may persist for several generations [9].

This chapter reviews briefly a selection of results of studies of the harm endured by relatives from alcohol abusers. It is concerned only with the close relatives living under the same roof as the excessive drinker and those most commonly affected, essentially members of the typical family unit – in other words, the drinker's children and partner. It deals with the categories of harm that have been the subject of most research to date and are the most serious for public health. Economic consequences and certain relational aspects are not considered. Although the division into distinct areas is consistent with most of the studies reviewed here, it is somewhat reductionist in the sense that it takes little account of the probably frequent interactions of those areas in reality.

CONSEQUENCES FOR CHILDREN

It is undeniable that children growing up in a family in which one or both parents have alcohol-related problems are at serious risk to their physical and mental health. Many guides, warnings, stories and other printed matter intended for the general public are published each year to highlight this. Publications of empirical studies of a scientific nature are less numerous, but the conclusions which may be drawn from these are more discriminating and may in some respects be less pessimistic than the categorical conclusions of certain popular or anecdotal publications [10]. Research with children of alcoholics has found that they suffered more often than other children from such problems as hyperactivity [11, 12], emotional disorders [13, 14], and behavioural difficulties [15, 16] and, later, from an increased propensity to abuse alcohol or other psychotropic substances [17, 18]. Once these associations were established, it proved very much more difficult to formulate valid generalizations about the mechanisms that might explain these correlations. A well-known difficulty is that the parents concerned, in addition to their alcohol-related problems, often suffer from other disorders of various kinds, which may also affect the children's health and state of mind.

Prenatal alcohol exposure

One major risk for the future development of the child is direct exposure to alcohol from maternal drinking during gestation. The indications are that the risk increases with the amount of alcohol consumed by the mother, but that it is also dependent on other factors, such as nutritional deficiency, smoking and the use of drugs, and genetic factors. The most serious form of impairment is fetal alcohol syndrome (FAS), characterized by serious damage to the central nervous system, growth defects and facial deformity [19]. It is conservatively estimated that, in Western countries, at least one child in 3000 is born with fetal alcohol syndrome [20]. Most estimates, however, often restricted to specific countries, report rates up to 10 times higher, of about 2 to 5 cases per 1000 births [4, 21, 22]. Other, less severe conditions, sometimes described as 'alcohol-related birth defects', are characterized in particular by learning and behavioural disorders. These impairments are estimated to be up to 10 times more common than fetal alcohol syndrome [23]. There is overwhelming evidence that prenatal alcohol exposure impairs child development seriously, possibly permanently. Severely affected cases, in particular, are considered unlikely to recover [24–26].

Abuse

Child abuse includes aspects as varied as physical violence, sexual abuse, abandonment, neglect or emotional abuse. In the United States, 4.7% of the child population are estimated to be victims of abuse [27]. Relatively few studies have examined closely the relationships between alcoholism and abuse. Research has so far not established a direct causal relationship, but has often confirmed correlations [28]. Thus, several investigations of the reasons for child abuse suggest that in a large proportion of families involved (ranging from 13% to more than 70%) the parents had substance-related problems, related mainly to drinking. Moreover, case reports indicate that most incidents of abuse occur when the parent or other abuser is under the influence of alcohol or other substances [29].

Family environment and psychological consequences

The family and social environment of the children of substance abusers is often chaotic and consequently not disposed to fostering balanced development. The children of alcohol abusers are liable to suffer emotional trauma which may affect their mental state. Velleman and Orford [30] in a study on the basis of recall of young adults found that, compared with a control group, the children of drinkers recalled many more negative experiences from their childhood. Their social life had been very limited and they had frequently been left to their own devices. They more often had to assume responsibilities inappropriate to their age, such as having to put one of their parents to bed or otherwise look after them. Also, they much more often remembered having been involved in parental disputes or having to keep secrets about a parent. Finally, many more than in the control group had been worried about the household's finances or had feared that their father would lose his job. Other studies of the conditions of children of parents with alcohol-related problems again have stressed the fragility of family cohesion (arguments, marital disruption, deaths) [31] or the inconsistent attitudes or behaviour of the parents [32].

As regards the possible psychological sequelae of such circumstances, it is necessary first to highlight the difficulty of distinguishing the possibly influencing factors. In his pioneering study on the 115 children (aged from 10 to 15 years) of alcoholics, Cork [33] found that 50 suffered from very serious, and 56 from fairly serious, emotional disorders. A more recent study, from New Zealand, of a cohort of 961 children compared the prevalence of psychiatric disorders diagnosed at the age of 15 years in children of alcohol-abusing parents with that of children of other parents [34]. The disorders studied (abuse/dependence, behavioural disorders, attention disorders/hyperactivity, affective and anxiety disorders) were between 2.2 and 3.9 times more common in the former than in the latter group, and these associations proved significant for all the disorders concerned. A notable outcome of this study was that, though multivariate analysis suggested influences of other prospectively measured parental variables (social status, religious belief, crime, psychiatric disorders, maternal addiction to smoking during pregnancy, and others), it in no way discounted the links established between the children's disorders and parental alcoholism.

The longitudinal study by Drake and Vaillant [35] of 174 sons of alcoholics, covered a much longer period (33 years) and indicated that disorders manifested in adolescence may subsequently disappear. Indeed, although these adolescents showed relational, emotional and medical disorders, as well as below average general skills, observations in adult life revealed no more personality disorders than in a comparative group from families without alcohol-related problems. Some studies on the long-term effects of parental alcoholism, however, reached a different conclusion: the target and control groups differed, particularly in respect of depression, anxiety, stress management or the occurrence of relational difficulties [36, 37]. In general, the results here again are mixed and preclude definitive conclusions about the outcome in adulthood of psychopathological risks to which children of alcoholic parents are exposed [10, 38].

Intergenerational transmission

Much of the research on children of parents with alcohol-related problems has concentrated on the issue of the risk of such children themselves becoming alcohol abusers in later life. The risk is not disputed, but estimates of its extent vary greatly, from two to ten times higher than for children of parents not affected [38]. These disparities may be explained by the use of different criteria of abuse and by other methodological differences [39]. In general, paternal alcoholism appears to be as much a determining factor for men as for women [40], whereas maternal alcoholism seems to affect women more specifically [41].

A number of etiological factors have been advanced to explain the intergenerational transmission of alcohol-related problems. Several studies suggest a genetically – thus not socially – transmitted vulnerability, though not as a sufficient condition [42–44]. Others indicate an environmentally induced vulnerability, due to a number of factors, including family influences specific to alcohol as well as indirect influences. Thus, parental behaviour and values in respect of alcohol are likely to have a modelling effect on future attitudes of children. Likewise, children may in the long term internalize parental expectations of the effects of alcohol (for example, relief of stress), which may influence their future behaviour in regard to alcohol [45]. Family risk-factors not specific to alcohol include those often associated with parental alcoholism (low cohesion of family, abuse or neglect of children, parental psychopathology). These may undermine the children in the long term, predisposing them from adolescence onwards to the use of alcohol or other psychotropic substances. Three groups of such factors may be distinguished: first, the different forms of co-morbidity observed in an alcoholic parents, such as antisocial personality disorder or depression [45]; second, as several studies have shown, such characteristics of the families of alcoholics as lack of family cohesion, a conflictual climate, violence, and lack of cognitive stimulation, which are correlated with the occurrence of alcohol-related problems in adolescence [18, 46] or with disorders known to be precursors of alcohol or drug abuse in adolescence [47]; and third, parental separation and divorce, common in families affected by an alcohol-related problem, which represent a considerable risk for the children concerned [48], particularly in relation to the occurrence of problems related to alcohol or other drugs [49, 50].

The factors contributing to intergenerational transmission do not act in isolation. Interactions, particularly between genetic and environmental factors, may considerably increase the risk of transmission. Thus, the recent work by Zucker and colleagues [47], based on longitudinal observations, suggests a marked interdependence of various risk factors, since different subtypes of affected families, resulting in different risk patterns for the children, could be recognized.

CONSEQUENCES FOR THE SPOUSE/PARTNER

Adults in the drinker's immediate circle (principally the spouse) differ fundamentally from children in that, in principle, they can call upon more resources for coping with the consequences. Adults may be expected to view the events with greater detachment than children and have more effective coping strategies. This in principle allows them to become more active in seeking solutions and means of protecting themselves. In practice, however, these theoretical abilities may be suppressed by the presence of various diseases or by emotionally inadequate responses, which may block any appropriate reaction on the part of the drinker's partner or induce prolonged confusion. Much of the literature on the spouses of drinkers concerns the controversial concept of 'co-dependence', described as a disorder specific to the drinker's spouse and contributing decisively to the establishment and preservation of the drinker's symptoms of alcoholic dependence [51, 52]. In this frame, however, we shall focus on two of the most frequently described types of consequences for the spouse of the excessive drinker: partner violence and marital disruption.

Partner violence

The possible link between marital violence and alcohol consumption has been the subject of much research since the 1970s. Several studies with reference groups suggest such a link. Thus, Rosenbaum and O'Leary [53] and Telch and Lindquist [54] showed that husbands of female victims of marital violence had a higher incidence of alcohol-related problems than non-violent spouses. Likewise, van Hasselt, Morrison and Bellack [55] showed that men who were violent towards a spouse scored significantly higher in the Michigan Alcoholism Screening Test (MAST) than men who were not. In addition, in a study of a sample of 484 male factory workers, Leonard et al. [56] found that 25% of workers who had pathological patterns of alcohol consumption also had violent marital disputes, whereas a markedly lower proportion of the same group of drinkers (13%; $p<0.01$) did not. The multivariate analyses undertaken in the study of Leonard et al. also suggest that demographic and psychosocial variables are not decisive in the relationship studied. In a study of a sample of 82 men released on licence, Miller [57] observed interactions between drinking and use of other drugs in relation to the frequency of violent acts against their spouses. Thus, it was only when no other psychotropic substances were taken that the frequency of such acts increased with increasing alcohol consumption. When the heavy drinker took cocaine, barbiturates or cannabis as well, the violent acts tended to decrease. More generally, the findings suggest a strong positive association between alcohol abuse and partner violence, except when large amounts of alcohol are taken. These findings may be explained by the anaesthetizing effect of alcohol taken in large quantities or with other substances [58].

Most studies refer to general drinking patterns rather than specifically to incidents of marital violence in relation to the degree of intoxication of the assailant at the time of an incident. The few event-centred studies carried out have found that a large proportion of assailants were under the influence of alcohol at the time of the event, ranging from 26% to 43%, depending on the studies [59–61]. A study reported by Leonard and Roberts [62] examined the interactions of young married couples (with or without a history of marital violence) by manipulating the effect of alcohol on the husband. The husbands received alcohol or alcohol-free drinks or a placebo (an apparently alcoholic beverage). The interactions when the husbands were under the influence of alcohol were markedly more often characterized by aggressive behaviour on the part of both husband and wife (criticism, disagreement, interruptions, etc.) than when they were given either alcohol-free drinks or placebo. The absence of a placebo effect, though the subjects were convinced they had taken as much alcohol as the target group, casts doubt on the hypothesis postulated by other authors of the importance of expectancies of the effects of alcohol in triggering violent acts [63].

Although these results overall show a link between drinking and marital violence, its nature is still difficult to determine. It seems that alcohol is never either a necessary or a sufficient condition for the occurrence of violent acts between spouses. In the current state of research, however, the correlations observed between alcohol and marital violence permit the formulation of certain basic hypotheses for explaining this link [64]. In the first place, as Leonard and Roberts [62] report and other similar experiments suggest, the psychotropic action of alcohol is likely to disinhibit the expression of certain aggressive tendencies. Secondly, other causes of spousal conflict associated with excessive use of alcohol may indirectly increase the risk of violence. Thirdly, the use of alcohol may simply be associated with antisocial attitudes or disorders that increase the risk of marital violence, with no necessary causal link to alcohol. These different paths should not be seen as alternatives – all may contribute to the correlation.

Although a direct effect of alcohol in inducing violent behaviour has not yet been established, everyday life points to such an effect and it is a matter of common belief and cultural expression – in songs, stories, and drama, for example. What should be stressed here is that the acceptance of the hypothesis of a direct psychotropic action of alcohol as an agent that promotes violence serves principally perpetrators of violent acts, who may indeed use alcohol sometimes to bring about acting out and sometimes to serve as an excuse to minimize their own responsibility for the violence. This aspect is important if it is realized that it is men who typically commit partner violence and that their victims are consequently typically women, as suggested by our recent study of telephone calls to a general helpline [65].

Break-up, divorce

We know of only a few studies that have examined the effects of problem drinking on marital cohesion. Aggregate-level studies suggest a bidirectional influence between divorce rates and alcohol consumption [66]. A few studies on the causes of marital breakdown indicate that excessive drinking by the husband is a ground of complaint commonly advanced by those concerned. Burns [67], for example, found that, of 16 factors examined as a cause of break-up, alcohol was in sixth position, and that 36% of women and 17% of men who were divorced or separated advanced alcohol as a reason. Some older studies also highlight its importance [68–70]. In a recent study of alcohol and marital life during the first year of marriage, Leonard and Roberts [71] noted a direct relationship between the mean daily consumption of alcohol by men and marital instability (separations, intended divorce), and that this relationship remained significant after testing for the effects of other variables (socio-demography, personality, hostile behaviour). By contrast, taking the mode of consumption in women as a basis, the same link could not be established in this study, although negative effects on the quality of the marriage were noted in both cases. More generally, the few available longitudinal studies from general population surveys suggest that heavy drinking contributes to divorce and, inversely, that divorce leads to an increase in alcohol consumption. Often, however, despite their prospective designs, these studies have long intervals between measurements (up to ten years in some cases) and may fail to detect the decisive steps of the process [72, 73].

In summary, despite the limited number of available studies – in particular, longitudinal studies with short intervals between measurements – it is generally accepted that excessive alcohol consumption is a cause of, or exacerbates, marital disputes and may result in the break-up of the couple or the family unit. To explain this deterioration in marital relations, the various consequences of the excessive drinking must be considered (difficulty in discharging responsibilities and duties, precarious employment, financial difficulties, poor social relations, unpredictable behaviour, aggressiveness, violence, sexual aggression towards the partner or children). Though the break-up of the marriage may be harmful, particularly to children, its preservation in such circumstances may also be harmful. In the longterm, therefore, the psychological stress experienced by the drinker's spouse may result in such disorders as loss of self-confidence, anxiety, or depression, which in turn may induce inappropriate responses to such stress (use of tranquillizers or even alcohol) [7].

CONCLUSION

Although in the current state of knowledge it is difficult to determine the extent of the suffering and harm undergone by the immediate family of the heavy drinker, it is likely to be considerable and at least as extensive – albeit different in nature – as that of the drinkers themselves.

Children are the most severely affected, since they can do little to protect themselves from the direct or indirect consequences of parental drinking. Some have already been severely and permanently scarred, even before they are exposed to parental behaviour. At least one child in 3000 in Western countries is born with fetal alcohol syndrome (FAS) and there is a ten-fold higher incidence of related disorders also linked to direct exposure to alcohol during gestation [23]. It is thus obvious that parental drinking can seriously harm a child's development, although its modes of action have only partially been elucidated. In particular, these involve abuse, neglect, isolation and insecurity or inconsistent parental behaviour and demands, which are much more common in the families of alcohol abusers than in others. Investigation of the long-term psychological effects of such harm in childhood has given somewhat contradictory findings, so that definitive conclusions cannot yet be drawn. What does seem well established, however, is that there is a substantial – two-fold to ten-fold – risk of intergenerational transmission of problem drinking. Several hypotheses have been advanced as regards modes of transmission, and recent studies by Zucker *et al.* [47] indicate that the aggregation of certain factors increases the risk.

The partners of alcohol-abusers also pay a heavy price. They are at serious risk of being subjected to violence, since marital violence is clearly more common with problem drinking. Although, so far, only hypothetical explanations have been advanced for marital violence in these circumstances, an alcohol-specific effect appears undeniable. Apart from the risk of marital violence, an alcohol-related problem may affect in other ways the quality of life and the health of the drinker's partner. The family is liable to split or to break up, as several studies of the causes of divorce have shown. A contrary condition, referred to as 'co-dependence' and described principally in the clinical literature, takes the form of a contradictory involvement on the part of the drinker's partner in maintaining the drinker's alcohol habit by efforts to conceal and compensate for it. In either case, and as regards such couples in general, the condition of the drinker's spouse or partner is liable to deteriorate, with consequent psychological or physical disorders.

This brief review suggests that the negative effects of excessive drinking on nondrinking family members, particularly on children, remain worrying and have to be considered as a relevant public health topic. Efforts designed to involve spouses or other family members in the treatment of the drinking patient are promising since they may have an impact not only on the immediate problems but also in preventing the enhanced risk of future addiction in the relatives of the drinking member.

REFERENCES

1. Appel, C. (1991) *Alkohol und Gesellschaft: Zur Relevanz und Aktualität der amerikanischen Temperenzbewegung*, Lambertus, Freiburg.
2. Clark, W.B. and Midanik, L. (1982) Alcohol use and alcohol problems among US adults: results of the 1979 survey, in National Institute on Alcohol Abuse and Alcoholism, ed.: *Alcohol and Health*, US Department of Health and Human Services, National Institute on Alcohol Abuse and Alcoholism, Rockville, MD, pp. 3–52 (Monograph 1).
3. Wilsnack, S.C., Wilsnack, R.W. and Klassen, A.D. (1986) Epidemiological research on women's drinking, 1978–1984, in National Institute on Alcohol Abuse and Alcoholism, ed.: *Women and Alcohol: Health Related Issue*, US Department of Health and Human Services, National Institute on Alcohol Abuse and Alcoholism, Rockville, MD, pp. 1–68 (Research Monograph 16).
4. Godfrey, C. (1994) Economic influences on change in population and personal substance behaviour, in *Addiction: Processes of Change* (eds G. Edwards and M. Lader), Oxford Medical Publications, Oxford, pp. 163–187.
5. Rice, N., Carr-Hill, R., Dixon, P. and Sutton, M. (1998) The influence of households on drinking behaviour: a multilevel analysis. *Social Science and Medicine* **46**(8), 971–979.
6. Leonard, K.E. and Rothbard, J.C. (1999) Alcohol and the marriage effect. *Journal of Studies on Alcohol* Suppl. No 13, 139–146.
7. Eurocare. (1998) *Alcohol Problems in the Family: A Report of the European Union*, Eurocare, St Ives, Cambridgeshire.
8. Nadeau, L. (1990) *Vivre avec l'alcool: la consommation, les effets, les abus* [Living with alcohol: consumption, consequences, misuse], Les Éditions de l'Homme, Montréal.
9. Miller, B.A. and Downs, W.R. (1993) The impact of family violence on the use of alcohol by women. *Alcohol World and Health Research* **17**(2), 137–143.
10. Barber, J.G. and Gilbertson, R. (1999) The drinker's children. *Substance Use and Misuse* **34**(3), 383–402.
11. Lund, C.A. and Landesman-Dwyer, S. (1979) Pre-delinquent and disturbed adolescents: the role of parental alcoholism, in *Currents in Alcoholism* (ed. M. Galanter), Grune and Stratton, New York, pp. 339–348.
12. Kuperman, S., Schlosser, S.S., Lidral, J. and Reich, W. (1999) Relationship of child psychopathology to parental alcoholism and antisocial personality disorder. *Journal of the American Academy of Child and Adolescent Psychiatry* **38**(6), 686–692.
13. Bennett, L.A., Wolin, S.J. and Reiss, D. (1988) Cognitive, behavioral, and emotional problems among school-age children of alcoholic parents. *American Journal of Psychiatry* **145**(2), 185–190.
14. Maynard, S. (1997) Growing up in an alcoholic family system: the effect on anxiety and differentiation of self. *Journal of Substance Abuse* **9**, 161–170.
15. Reich, W., Earls, F., Frankel, O. and Shayka, J.J. (1993) Psychopathology in children of alcoholics. *Journal of the American Academy of Child Psychiatry* **32**, 995–1002.
16. Johnson, J.L. and Leff, M. (1999) Children of substance abusers: overview of research findings. *Pediatrics* **103**(5 Pt 2), 1085–1099.
17. Reich, W. (1997) Prospective studies of children of alcoholic parents. *Alcohol Health and Research World* **21**(3), 255–257.
18. Sher, K.J. (1991) *Children of Alcoholics: A Critical Appraisal of Theory and Research*, The University of Chicago Press, Chicago.

19. Larkby, C. and Day, N. (1997) The effects of prenatal alcohol exposure. *Alcohol Health and Research World* **21**(3), 192–198.
20. Abel, E.L. and Sokol, R.J. (1991) A revised conservative estimate of the incidence of FAS and its economic impact. *Alcoholism: Clinical and Experimental Research* **15**, 514–524.
21. Little, B.B., Snell, L.H., Rosenfeld, C.R., Gilstrap, L.C. III and Gant, N.F. (1990) Failure to recognize fetal alcohol syndrome in newborn infants. *American Journal of Diseases of Children* **144**, 1142–1164.
22. Sampson, P.D., Streissguth, A.P., Bookstein, F.L. et al. (1997) Incidence of fetal alcohol syndrome and prevalence of alcohol-related neurodevelopmental disorder [see comments]. *Teratology* **56**(5), 317–326.
23. Robertson, B.E. (1993) *Alcohol Disabilities Primer: a Guide to Physical and Psychosocial Disabilities Caused by Alcohol Use*, CRC Press, Boca Raton/Ann Arbor/London/Tokyo.
24. Stromland, K. and Hellstrom, A. (1996) Fetal alcohol syndrome – an ophthalmological and socioeducational prospective study. *Pediatrics* **97**(6 Pt 1), 845–850.
25. Steinhausen, H.C. and Spohr, H.L. (1998) Long-term outcome of children with fetal alcohol syndrome: psychopathology, behavior, and intelligence. *Alcoholism: Clinical and Experimental Research* **22**(2), 334–338.
26. Loser, H., Bierstedt, T. and Blum, A. (1999) [Fetal alcohol syndrome in adulthood. A long-term study]. *Deutsche Medizinische Wochenschrift* **124**(14), 412–418.
27. Wang, C.T. and Daro, D. (1998) *Current Trends in Child Abuse Reporting and Fatalities: The Results of the 1997 Annual Fifty State Survey*, National Committee to Prevent Child Abuse, Chicago, IL.
28. Young, N.K. (1997) Effects of alcohol and other drugs on children. *Journal of Psychoactive Drugs* **29**(1), 23–42.
29. Magura, S. and Laudet, A.B. (1996) Parental substance abuse and child maltreatment: review and implications for intervention. *Children and Youth Services Review* **18**(3), 193–220.
30. Velleman, R. and Orford, J. (1990) Young adult offspring of parents with drinking problems: recollections of parents' drinking and its immediate effects. *British Journal of Clinical Psychology* **29**(3), 297–317.
31. Orford, J. (1990) Alcohol and the family: an international review of the literature with implications for research and practice, in *Research Advances in Alcohol and Drug Problems* (eds L.T. Kozlowski, H.M. Annis, H.D. Cappell, et al.), Plenum Press, New York/London, pp. 81–155.
32. West, M.O. and Prinz, R.J. (1987) Parental alcoholism and childhood psychopathology. *Psychological Bulletin* **102**(2), 204–218.
33. Cork, R.M. (1969) *The Forgotten Children*, Alcoholism and Drug Addiction Research Foundation, Toronto.
34. Lynskey, M.T., Fergusson, D.M. and Horwood, L.J. (1994) The effect of parental alcohol problems on rates of adolescent psychiatric disorders. *Addiction* **89**, 1277–1286.
35. Drake, R.E. and Vaillant, G.E. (1988) Predicting alcoholism and personality disorder in a 33-year longitudinal study of children of alcoholics. *British Journal of Addiction* **83**, 799–807.
36. Black, C., Bucky, S.F. and Wilder-Padilla, S. (1986) The interpersonal and emotional consequences of being an adult child of an alcoholic. *The International Journal of the Addictions* **21**(2), 213–231.
37. Belliveau, J.M. and Stoppard, J.M. (1995) Parental alcohol abuse and gender as predictors of psychopathology in adult children of alcoholics. *Addictive Behaviors* **20**(5), 619–625.

38. Sher, K.J. (1997) Psychological characteristics of children of alcoholics. *Alcohol Health and Research World* **21**(3), 247–254.
39. Windle, M. (1997) Concepts and issues in COA research. *Alcohol Health and Research World* **21**(3), 185–191
40. Jennison, K.M. and Johnson, K.A. (1998) Alcohol dependence in adult children of alcoholics: longitudinal evidence of early risk. *Journal of Drug Education* **28**(1), 19–37.
41. Pollock, V.E., Schneider, L.S., Gabrielli, W.F. and Goodwin, D.W. (1987) Sex of parent and offspring in the transmission of alcoholism: a meta-analysis. *Journal of Nervous and Mental Disease* **173**, 668–673.
42. Light, J.M., Irvine, K.M. and Kjerulf, L. (1996) Estimating genetic and environmental effects of alcohol use and dependence from a national survey: a 'quasi-adoption' study. *Journal of Studies on Alcohol* **57**(5), 507–520.
43. Sigvardsson, S., Bohman, M. and Cloninger, C.R. (1996) Replication of the Stockholm Adoption Study of alcoholism. Confirmatory cross-fostering analysis. *Archives of General Psychiatry* **53**(8), 681–687.
44. McGue, M. (1997) A behavioral-genetic perspective on children of alcoholics. *Alcohol Health and Research World* **21**(3), 210–217.
45. Ellis, D.A., Zucker, R.A. and Fitzgerald, H.E. (1997) The role of family influences in development and risk. *Alcohol Health and Research World* **21**(3), 218–226.
46. Johnson, V. and Pandina, R. (1991) Effects of the family environment on adolescent substance use, delinquency and coping styles. *American Journal of Drug and Alcohol Abuse* **17**, 71–88.
47. Zucker, R.A., Ellis, D.A., Bingham, C.R. and Fitzgerald, H.E. (1996) The development of alcoholic subtypes: risk variation among alcoholic families during the early childhood years. *Alcohol Health and Research World* **20**, 46–54.
48. Neighbors, B.D., Forehand, R. and Bau, J.J. (1997) Interparental conflict and relations with parents as predictors of young adult functioning. *Development and Psychopathology* **9**(1), 169–187.
49. Wills, T.A., Mariani, J. and Filer, M. (1996) The role of family and peer relationships in adolescent substance use, in *Handbook of Social Support and the Family* (eds G.R. Pierce, B.R. Sarason and I.G. Sarason), Plenum Press, New York, pp. 521–549.
50. Wolfinger, N.H. (1998) The effects of parental divorce on adult tobacco and alcohol consumption. *Journal of Health and Social Behavior* **39**(3), 254–269.
51. Holmila, M. (1997) Family roles and being a problem drinker's intimate other. *European Addiction Research* **3**(1), 37–42.
52. Treadway, D. (1990) Codependency: disease, metaphor or fad? *Family Therapy Networker* **14**(1), 39–42.
53. Rosenbaum, A. and O'Leary, K.D. (1981) Children: the unintended victims of marital violence. *American Journal of Orthopsychiatry* **51**, 692–699.
54. Telch, C. and Lindquist, C. (1984) Violent versus nonviolent couples: a comparison of patterns. *Psychotherapy* **21**, 242–248.
55. Van Hasselt, V.B., Morrison, R.L. and Bellack, A.S. (1985) Alcohol use in wife abusers and their spouses. *Addictive Behaviors* **10**, 127–135.
56. Leonard, K.E., Bromen, E.J., Parkinson, D.K., Day, N.L. and Ryan, C.M. (1985) Patterns of alcohol use and physically aggressive behavior. *Journal of Studies on Alcohol* **46**, 279–282.
57. Miller, B.A. (1990) The interrelationships between alcohol and drugs and family violence, in *Drugs and Violence: Causes, Correlates, and Consequences* (eds M. De La Rosa, E.Y. Lambert and B. Gropper), US Department of Health and Human Services, Rockville, MD, National Institute on Drug Abuse, pp. 177–207 (NIDA Research Monograph 103).

58. Yegidis, B.L. (1992) Family violence: contemporary research findings and practice issues. *Community Mental Health Journal* **28**, 519–530.
59. Gayford, J.J. (1975) Wife battering: a preliminary study of 100 cases. *British Medical Journal* **1**, 194–197.
60. Dobash, R.E. and Dobash, R.P. (1987) Violence toward wives, in *Coping with Disorder in the Family* (ed. J. Orford), Croom Helm, London, pp. 608–622 (2).
61. Pernanen, K. (1991) *Alcohol in Human Violence*, Guilford Press, New York.
62. Leonard, K.E. and Roberts, L.J. (1996) Alcohol in the early years of marriage. *Alcohol Health and Research World* **20**(3), 192–196.
63. Kreutzer, J.S., Schneider, H.G. and Myatt, C.R. (1984) Alcohol, aggression and assertiveness in men: dosage and expectancy effects. *Journal of Studies on Alcohol* **45**(3), 275–278.
64. Holtzworth-Munroe, A., Bates, L., Smutzler, N. and Sandin, E. (1997) A brief review of the research on husband violence. 1. Maritally violent versus nonviolent men. *Aggression and Violent Behavior* **2**(1), 65–99.
65. Maffli, E. and Bahner, U. (1999) *Domestic Violence and Alcohol in Helpline Calls*, Paper presented at the 25th Annual Alcohol Epidemiology Symposium of the Kettil Bruun Society, Montreal.
66. Caces, M.F., Harford, T.C., Williams, G.D. and Hanna, E.Z. (1999) Alcohol consumption and divorce rates in the United States. *Journal of Studies on Alcohol* **60**(5), 647–652.
67. Burns, A. (1984) Perceived causes of marriage breakdown and conditions of life. *Journal of Marriage and the Family* **46**, 551–562.
68. Straus, R. and Bacon, S.D. (1951) Alcoholism and social stability: a study of occupational integration in 2023 male clinic patients. *Quarterly Journal of Studies on Alcohol* **12**, 231–260.
69. Levinger, G. (1966) Sources of marital dissatisfaction among applicants for divorce. *American Journal of Orthopsychiatry* **36**, 803-807.
70. Hedri, A. (1971) [Marital crises in prosperous families]. *Zeitschrift für Psychotherapie und medizinische Psychologie* **21**, 35–38.
71. Leonard, K.E. and Roberts, L.J. (1998) Marital aggression, quality, and stability in the first year of marriage: findings from the Buffalo Newlywed Study, in *The Developmental Course of Marital Dysfunction* (ed. T.N. Bradbury), Cambridge University Press, New York, pp. 44–73.
72. Romelsjö, A., Lazarus, N.B., Kaplan, G.A. and Cohen, R.D. (1991) The relationship between stressful life situations and changes in alcohol consumption in a general population sample. *British Journal of Addiction* **86**(2), 157–169.
73. Power, C., Rodgers, B. and Hope, S. (1999) Heavy alcohol consumption and marital status: disentangling the relationship in a national study of young adults. *Addiction* **94**(10), 1477–1487.

Chapter seven

Accidents, suicide and violence

I. Rossow, K. Pernanen and J. Rehm

INTRODUCTION

Whether external trauma is classified as accident, suicide (or suicide attempt) or violence is determined by the characteristics of those who caused it and their acts and intentions. Unintentional injury to oneself and others is classified as accident, intentional injury to oneself as suicidal behaviour, and intentional injury to others as violence. These distinctions are linked to ideas about social responsibility and its apportionment in relation to injury or fatal outcome. In all three categories the injury may be the same but the social consequences differ in important respects. This is reflected in the social reactions to the three forms of trauma.

In Western countries, automobile accidents are the form of external trauma responsible for the largest proportion of fatalities, usually followed by other types of accident, and suicide and homicide. The following distribution of causes of death from accidents was found in a United States national database with over 150 000 fatalities from external trauma: motor vehicle collisions 32%; falls 9%; fire 4%; drowning 4%; industrial accidents 3%; and poisoning 3% [1]. Thus, more than half of deaths from trauma were due to accidents. Suicide accounted for 18% and homicide for 13%. The relative incidence of the different forms of external trauma varies among different societies. In European countries, in general, motor vehicle collisions and homicide account for a smaller proportion of deaths from external trauma than in the United States. In Finland, for instance, homicide accounts for a much smaller proportion of deaths from external trauma, and suicide for a higher proportion [2], than in the United States. In sub-Saharan Africa, falls are the commonest cause of fatal injury, followed by road-traffic injury, assault, burns and poisoning [3]. Internal shifts

---

Harald Klingemann and Gerhard Gmel (eds.), Mapping the Social Consequences of Alcohol Consumption, 93–112.
© *2001 Kluwer Academic Publishers. Printed in Great Britain.*

between the categories also occur in the same country over time [4]. In most societies, men, especially young men, die much more often than women from external trauma.

ALCOHOL AND EXTERNAL TRAUMA

Alcohol use increases the risk of injury in many forms of external trauma, including traffic accidents, falls and other household accidents, fire, sports and recreational accidents, suicidal behaviour, and interpersonal violence [5–12]. Evidence indicates also that alcohol in the body at the time of injury is associated with greater severity of injury [13, 14].

Wechsler et al. [15], in their emergency-room study, found that 17% of the patients tested positive for breath-alcohol – 24% of the injury victims and 10% of the others. For categories of external trauma, the proportions were as follows: accidents, 22%; transport accidents (mostly automobile accidents), 30%; domestic accidents, 22%; occupational accidents, 16%; and fights and assault, 54%.

In about 50% of the accident victims and 71% of the assault and fight victims who had been drinking prior to the trauma, the blood-alcohol concentration (BAC) was at least 0.05 g/100 ml. Of the accident victims who had been drinking, 32% of the occupational accident group – the lowest proportion – were at this blood-alcohol-concentration level.

Walsh and Macleod [16] in their study of hospital emergency cases in Scotland also found that 70% of the victims of violence, by far the highest proportion, had a positive BAC, compared with 10% of the combined group of victims of traffic, home, work and sports accidents. Cases of injury from assault also showed a high proportion with levels of 0.08 g/100 ml or higher. Recalculations of the material show that although assault victims formed only 7% of the total sample they made up 28% of the cases with a positive alcohol test. Similar findings are common in the more recent literature. A Canadian emergency-room study by Macdonald et al. [17] found that 42% of patients with injuries from violence had a blood-alcohol concentration of over 0.08 g/100 ml compared with 4% of those with injuries from accidents.

Thus, while the proportion of victims of violence may be relatively lower than that of accident victims in general external-trauma samples, it is much higher when trauma victims who had been drinking are included, and higher again with the inclusion of relatively highly intoxicated victims of trauma. Clearly, the contribution of alcohol-related violence to health and social consequences of external trauma is higher than that of other causes of injury.

ALCOHOL AND ACCIDENTS

A long series of retrospective studies using a case–control design has compared BAC levels in individuals who had been in a collision or suffered trauma with those of selected individuals who had not had trauma [5, 10–13, 18]. Most of these studies used the emergency room for controls and established associations between BAC levels and accidents and injuries as a whole, as well as between BAC levels and most sub-categories of accidents and injuries. The associations are not equally strong for all of these categories. Several studies indicate, for example, that alcohol is more strongly associated with accidental drowning [19, 20]; around half of the cases of accidental drowning are attributable to alcohol, compared with a significantly lower proportion of victims of sports and domestic accidents [5, 21]. Stinson and DeBakey [22] also found that fractions of various categories of fatal injury attributable to alcohol varied with type of injury.

The relation between alcohol intake and traffic accidents has been that most studied in these respects. Here one of the most influential case–control series has been the Grand Rapids (USA) study of 5985 traffic collisions [11, 23]. Further analysis of that study indicates that all levels of BAC are associated with an increased risk of motor vehicle crashes, relative to a BAC of zero, and an accelerating slope on which the risk of injury increases markedly with high BAC [11]. Another case–control study in the United States, which combined data from a fatal-accident reporting system [24], reported an almost twofold relative risk for a BAC of 0.02 g/100 ml (relative to zero), increasing to ninefold with a BAC in the range of 0.05 g/100 ml to 0.09 g/100 ml.

Related lines of research include BAC studies of patients seen in emergency rooms, and the reports of coroners [12, 25]. Although the prevalence of positive BACs varies considerably among injured individuals, the literature generally shows a positive correlation between trauma risk and BAC, with no clear indication of a threshold effect.

Alcohol is related to all forms of accident, but the strength of its relationship with categories of accident is variable. As workplace accidents incur high social costs [26, see also Chapter 5 in this volume] they are considered next.

Studies of occupational accidents and injuries in the workplace have generally demonstrated only a relatively small involvement of alcohol. Self-reported drinking at work varies considerably among countries and types of workplace, and although it is generally assumed to be unusual, as for instance in the study of Wiebe et al. [27], where 5% of a general population sample reported workplace drinking, it has also been found that a fourth of a workplace sample reported drinking at work in the previous year [28]. Additionally, hangovers and drinking just before work may contribute to alcohol-related workplace problems, but Ames et al. [28] did not find that they contributed significantly to workplace accidents. The risk of workplace accidents has been found to be higher among self-reported problem-drinkers than among others [29], and it increases with increasing level of drinking [30].

The extent to which workplace injuries and fatalities are alcohol-related (in the sense that BAC was positive or above 0.05 g/100 ml) varies greatly. Thus, Shannon and co-workers [31] reported that alcohol levels 'likely to produce impairment' was found in 2% of fatal occupational accidents; Wechsler et al. [15] found that 5% of emergency-room patients injured at work had a positive BAC, above 0.05 g/100 ml; and according to Hollo et al. [32] BACs exceeded this level in 11% of workplace fatalities in Australia; whereas Gutierrez-Fisac et al. [30] reported that 17% of occupational accidents were attributable to alcohol, and Naranjo and Bremner [33] that 'at least 22% of work-related accidents may have involved alcohol use'. These variations probably reflect differences in the methods used in the various studies, but most likely also differences among countries and workplaces with respect to drinking just before or at work.

Drinking patterns and accidents

A number of studies have demonstrated that heavy drinkers and alcohol abusers are at significantly increased risk of fatal accidents [34–36], and, at the aggregate level, that an increase in total alcohol consumption, which implies an increase in the number of heavy-drinking occasions as well as in proportions of heavy drinkers, is followed by an increase in fatal accidents [37, 38].

Studies relating usual drinking patterns or levels to risk of injury have found the risk of accidents to be positively related to increasing average-intake levels, and to increase at relatively low volumes of intake [39]. Such studies have also highlighted the importance of specific drinking-pattern variables in modifying the association between total intake and risk of injury. Both frequent heavy drinking and frequent subjective drunkenness are associated with injury, particularly injury from violence [40]. Frequency of heavy drinking has also been associated with a greater likelihood of death from injury, relative to other causes [41]. Wells and MacDonald [42] found, however, that the association between drinking pattern and car collisions, work accidents and sports accidents was significant only in the younger age groups (15–24 years and 25–34 years). One important line of research in this area has empirically defined a variable of usual drinking pattern that is most closely associated with the risk of injury and drunk-driving behaviour after adjusting for other drinking-pattern variables and characteristics of the drinker [43–46]. Greatest risk is found to be associated with variance in drinking, or approximately the statistical variance in the amount consumed by an individual across different drinking occasions for that individual. This variance term reaches its highest value in individuals who consume relatively large amounts on some occasions, and whose highest amounts are markedly greater than their average amount per occasion. Overall, the available literature relating usual drinking patterns to risk of injury indicates a positive association with total dose, and a stronger association with occasions of relatively heavy drinking.

Comparisons of the impact of alcohol on accidents across drinking cultures indicate that alcohol is involved in a larger fraction of accidents in relatively 'dry' countries or cultures than in 'wetter' areas. Cherpitel [47] found that fatality rates of alcohol-related injuries were higher in a county in which per capita consumption was low than in a county in which it was high. In line with this, Skog [38] has found on the basis of time series analyses of 14 European countries that the relative impact of per capita consumption on fatal accidents is higher in the northern countries, which are characterized by 'dryness' and 'explosive' drinking patterns, and that the attributable fraction also is somewhat higher in these countries than in the 'wetter', Mediterranean countries.

In summary, the evidence reviewed above indicates that the amount consumed per occasion and, more specifically, blood-alcohol concentration, are the critical factors in determining risk of accidental injury. The degree of risk for accidents will depend also upon the setting, the requirements of the situation for high-order psychomotor skills, and how experienced the individual is.

Acute intoxication: processes determining the relationship between alcohol and accidents

Controlled experimental studies have demonstrated that cognitive and psychomotor effects of moderate doses of alcohol – on reaction time, cognitive processing, coordination and vigilance – affect risk of injury [12, 48–50]. Several reviews have indicated how low to moderate doses of alcohol affect psychomotor skills used in driving [48–52]. A common purpose of many of these reviews was to assess evidence relevant to establishing legal limits on BAC for drink-driving legislation [53].

An earlier review [48] of 41 studies of reaction time in relation to doses of ethanol found that 14 showed performance deficits at BACs of 0.05 g/100 ml or less, and only two failed to show an effect at 0.06 g/100 ml or more. Generally, effects of cognitive impairment on, for example, performance on divided attention tasks appeared variably in the range of 0.05 g/100 ml to 0.08 g/100 ml [48]. More recently, Krüger and co-workers reviewing 220 experimental studies of the effects of alcohol administration on psychophysical functions (such as vision or psychomotor function), automatic processing and control actions [49] found subtle effects on vision at very low doses, of around 0.03 g/100 ml, and on visual skills needed to assess depth and motion at doses above 0.05 g/100 ml. Automatic processing deficits typically showed a threshold at around 0.05 g/100 ml and increased steadily above this level. The review by Eckardt and colleagues [50] concluded that the threshold dose for negative effects on psychomotor tasks is generally found around 0.04 g/100 ml to 0.05 g/100 ml and also stated, 'injury can occur as a result of alcohol's disruption of psychomotor function in individuals at BACs of approximately 10 mM' (p. 1015), which is equivalent to slightly less than 0.05 g/100 ml.

The extent of psychomotor impairment varies according to the experience of the individual, and learning reduces the adverse impact on performance [54]. Analysis of the Grand Rapids data [55] showed that the risk of motor vehicle crashes increased more with increasing BAC level of the infrequent drinkers than of the more frequent, and thus more experienced, drinkers (Figure 1).

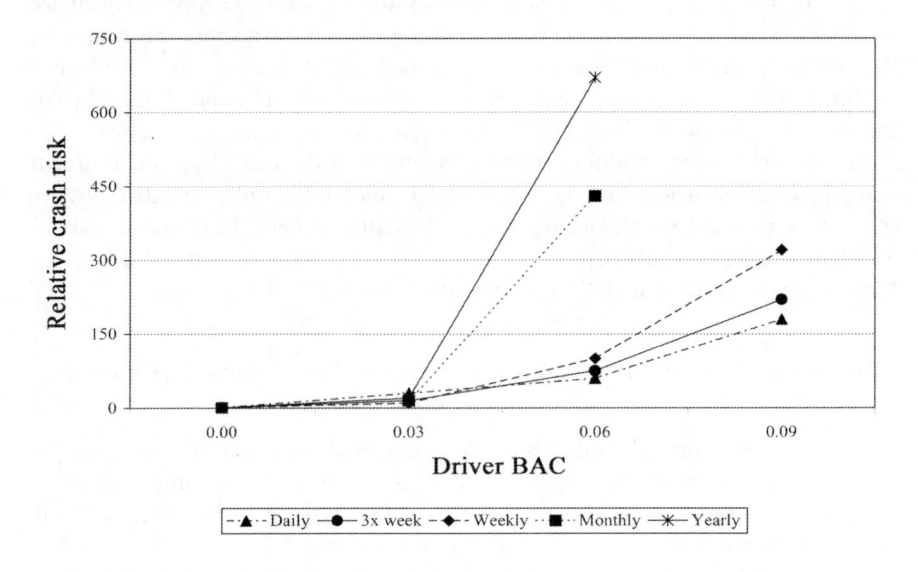

Figure 1 Road traffic crashes: driver BAC and relative crash risk plotted separately for different drinking frequencies. Grand Rapids data, – reanalysed. US National data. (based on National Highway Traffic Safety Administration, (1992) cited in Edwards *et al.* [55].

In sum, at above 0.04 g/100 ml alcohol impairs cognitive and psychomotor functions. Below that level it may have positive effects on some tasks [50, 56], although the empirical evidence is still scarce. These are overall effects, which vary with genetic predisposition and personal characteristics, as well as with the situational characteristics (e.g. alcohol consumption with a meal).

SUICIDE AND PARASUICIDE

Numerous studies have demonstrated significant associations between alcohol consumption and suicidal behaviour – both completed suicide and intentional self-inflicted injury. Heavy drinking or alcohol abuse is a major risk factor for suicide and attempted suicide: heavy drinkers commit about one fifth of male suicides [57], and around 5% of male alcohol abusers take their own lives [58, 59]. The risk of suicide increases significantly with level of alcohol consumption

[60], and for heavy drinkers it is some 2 to 20 times higher than for others [61 for a review]. Reports indicate that significant proportions (10% to 50%) of suicide attempters (parasuicide) admitted to hospital were heavy drinkers [62–66], and that in the Nordic countries around half of those admitted were under the influence of alcohol at the time of the attempt [67]. Population studies have also demonstrated a significant association between alcohol consumption and self-reported parasuicide, the proportion of parasuicides increasing significantly with level of alcohol consumption or frequency of intoxication (Figure 2) [68, 69]. Also at the aggregate level, male suicide rates co-vary with total alcohol consumption, changing immediately and significantly in response to change in total alcohol consumption [61 for a review]. In general, these studies have suggested that an increase of one litre in total consumption raises male suicide rates by from 2.5% to 15%, but does not significantly change female rates. In studies of possible beverage-specific effects of alcohol consumption on suicide rates, Gruenewald et al. [70] found that in the United States beer was the beverage most strongly associated with suicide rates; and Norström and Rossow [71] showed that in both Sweden and Norway suicide rates were influenced by consumption of spirits, but only in Norway by beer.

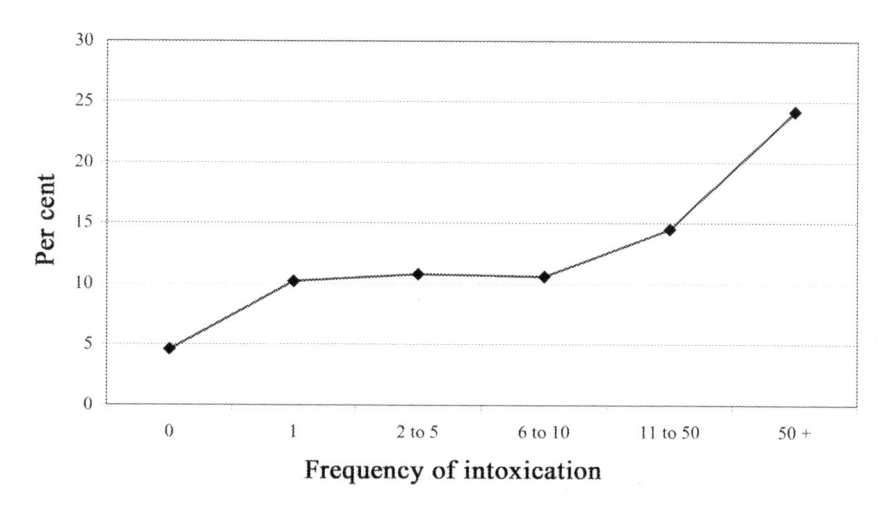

Figure 2 Life-time prevalence of attempted suicide among 12–19-year-old students by frequency of intoxication in the past year [Source: 69].

Given that total consumption and proportion of heavy drinkers are higher for men than for women, it is not surprising that a larger proportion of men than of women who commit or attempt suicide are heavy drinkers [65, 72, 73]. The risk among heavy drinkers appears to be of the same magnitude for both sexes [74–76], indicating that heavy drinking not only increases the risk of suicidal behaviour but also outweighs the significant overall sex differences in such behaviour. More research is needed in this area, given particularly the sex differences in psychiatric co-morbidity of heavy drinkers [77].

Comparison of the impact of alcohol consumption on suicide across drinking cultures has demonstrated that the relative effect tends to be rather less in 'wet' countries, such as France [78] and Portugal [79], than in 'dry' countries, such as Sweden [78, 80] and Norway [73]. The explanation may be that social marginalization and stigmatization of heavy drinkers are less in 'wet' cultures, but also that the more 'explosive' drinking patterns tend to characterize the 'drier' cultures [61, 78].

There are three possible explanations of the observed association between drinking and suicidal behaviour: (a) the long-term effects of heavy drinking may be a causal factor in suicidal behaviour because of their action on the serotonergic system, leading, for instance, to secondary depression, social disintegration, personal loss; (b) the association may to some extent be spurious – some individuals may be predisposed to both heavy drinking and suicidal behaviour, owing to, for instance, primary depression or personality traits; (c) episodes of acute intoxication may trigger suicidal impulses and injuries by reinforcing a depressive mood and removing inhibitions to self-hurting. The extent to which these explanations are valid, or what their relative weight would be, is most uncertain.

In summary, there is much empirical evidence that alcohol plays a significant part in suicidal behaviour, whether fatal or not, and that both acute intoxication and chronic abuse increase the risk of intentional self-harm.

ALCOHOL AND VIOLENCE

In the study of injury and death from trauma the focus is naturally on alcohol use by the victim. In suicide, only the victim is immediately relevant, and in many accidents also; relatively often, of course, the trauma is caused by the carelessness or negligence of others. Traffic accidents caused by drunken drivers are the most obvious example of this, but injuries and fatalities to others, unrelated to traffic, are also caused by actions or lack of action on the part of intoxicated individuals.

In relation to violence the focus of responsibility and explanation is placed mostly on the perpetrator. Victims are easier to locate than perpetrators, however, and there is more detailed knowledge about the use of alcohol by victims of violence and the influence of alcohol, mainly from emergency-room studies and coroners' inquests. Perpetrators, if they are arrested, are most easily found in jails and prisons, sometimes long after the violent episode, and a few surveys of the relationship between alcohol and violence have been carried out on such populations. Other studies of violent events are based on police reports and court documents.

Aggregate-level studies

Many countries keep relatively exact statistics on the sale of alcohol. Sales generally reflect the consumption levels sufficiently well to be used in *time series analyses* of the relation of per capita consumption of alcohol to rates of violent crime. Lenke [81] found that countries varied greatly in the closeness of this relationship. Among the five countries studied by Lenke, Finland showed the closest relationship between variation in alcohol sales and variation in volume of violent crime. Denmark and France showed little or no relationship, and in Sweden and Norway the relationships were relatively strong. In line with this, recent time series analyses of alcohol sales and homicide rates in 14 European countries demonstrated that the impact of alcohol consumption on homicide was highest in the most northern countries (Finland, Sweden and Norway) and weakest in the Mediterranean countries (Italy, France, Spain and Portugal); estimates for the other EU-countries of central Europe were intermediate [82].

Sudden changes in the availability of alcohol are sometimes related to changes in legislation, such as when beer or wine is introduced in grocery stores, or the age limit for alcohol purchase is raised or lowered. Strikes of employees of liquor stores or others in the alcohol distribution chain also give rise to such 'natural experiments'. On the whole, studies show that relatively sudden decreases in alcohol availability lead to lower levels of, at least, trauma from violence and accidents, fewer victims of violence presenting at emergency rooms, and fewer incidents of violent crime coming to the attention of the authorities. This occurred, for instance, subsequent to the anti-alcohol campaign in the USSR during the Gorbachev era, when alcohol sales fell significantly [83]. The opposite generally occurs when availability and consumption increase, as during the 1990s in the former Soviet republics of Estonia [84] and Russia [85].

Studies of violent episodes

We have seen that a larger proportion of victims of violence had been drinking at the time of injury than of victims of most other types of external trauma. Several Norwegian studies, specifically on injury from violence, also found a high proportion of drinking victims. Dahl *et al.* [86] found that more than two thirds of male and more than half of female victims of violence were under the influence of alcohol on admission to a hospital surgery ward in Stavanger, Norway. Two other studies in Norway, in Oslo in 1994 and Bergen in 1994/1995, found 64% and 69%, respectively, of those presenting at an emergency department with injuries from violence to be under the influence [87, 88]; only 1.3% of the patients in the Bergen study were presenting with injuries from violence. Danish studies put the proportion at 3–4% [89].

Studies of violent crime, based on *police reports* and *court documents* pertaining to the incident, have found similar proportions of drinking victims of violence

[90 for a review]. In addition to the relatively high blood-alcohol levels of injuries from violence found in emergency-room studies, several autopsy studies indicate that homicide victims who had been drinking had high levels of alcohol in their blood at the time of death [91, 92].

The intoxication of the victim is of special interest to the health-care system, in part because this information is needed for a valid diagnosis of brain injury and to provide proper care. The drinking of the perpetrator is of interest to the legal system. It is of interest also from a research perspective. As with findings from time series analyses of levels of alcohol consumption and rates of violent crime, countries show consistent differences in the proportions of violent-crime offenders who were under the influence of alcohol at the time of a crime. On the basis of studies selected as being sufficiently representative of a jurisdiction or geographical area and with sufficiently large sample-sizes, the following rough generalizations may be made about those proportions: Sweden, 70–80%; Norway, 70–75%; Finland, 60–70%; the United States, 55–60% and Canada 30–45%. These figures are probably contaminated to some extent by the attention given to alcohol as a cause of violence in a country and the related care with which drinking by those involved in violence is reported and recorded [93].

Interviews conducted with prisoners in North America have shown the same high proportions of offenders who had been drinking before the violent crime. In a United States study, 53% of federal prisoners who had committed homicide reported prior drinking, while 55% and 62%, respectively, of inmates convicted of manslaughter and aggravated assault reported the same [94]. In a Canadian study of newly admitted federal prisoners, the proportions of homicide and of assault offenders who had been drinking were, respectively, 50% and 60% [95]. This study also showed that the concurrent use of other psychoactive drugs is common in violent crime, which makes it difficult to determine the causal role of alcohol. (The same multi-use problem is increasingly evident also in the study of some accidents – traffic accidents, in particular) [96].

Studies of drinking patterns and risk of violence

As both violence and drinking pattern have become subjects of epidemiological investigation, it has become increasingly common to study how patterns of alcohol consumption are related to risk of injury and participation in violence. Rossow [97] reports from a study of 2711 Norwegians from the general population that the risk of having been in a fight after drinking increased with frequency of drinking, frequency of being intoxicated and frequency of visiting public drinking places (Figure 3). Survey studies in other countries have reported similar dose-response patterns.

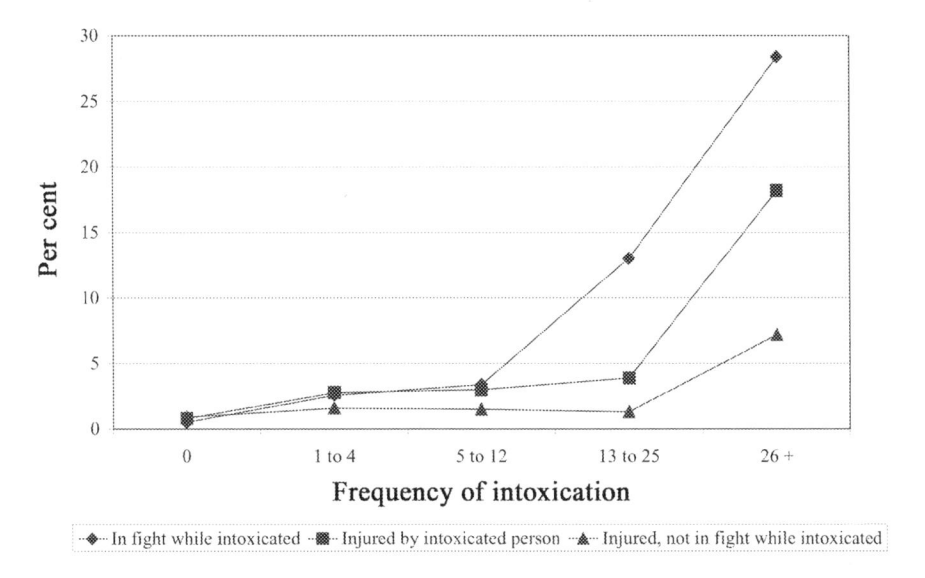

Figure 3 Proportion of respondents in a national survey (in Norway, 1994) reporting having been in a fight while intoxicated during the past year, by frequency of intoxication during the past year [Source: 97].

Studies of drinking events

The risk of being arrested at high levels of intoxication is likely to be greater than at lower levels, and estimates of the prevalence of intoxicated offenders can, therefore, become elevated in violent-crime samples. It is important, therefore, to use other data to study events of violence. This is done in part by using emergency-room samples. Such samples, however, are also subject to selection bias [98]. The Canadian community study mentioned earlier [90] found that drinking had occurred prior to 54% of relatively mild types of violent episode, of which 11% needed medical attention for injuries and in 15% of which police were involved. This indicates that alcohol is involved also in a high proportion of violence that does not come to the attention of the police or the health care system.

Several explanations have been suggested for the high risk of violence in connection with alcohol consumption:

(1) Pharmacological effects of alcohol may directly increase the risk of aggressive behaviour. Alcohol may be a 'disinhibitor' which releases aggressive tendencies that are inhibited in the sober state. This explanation seems to be little more than a summary of observed behaviour of some people after drinking in certain circumstances.

(2) Alcohol may affect vigilance, attention and cognitive processing, and the intoxicated person focuses on the immediate situation. Attention is confined largely to the 'here-and-now', with a consequent tendency for emotional instability. Drinkers shunt aside the wider social context and disregard the longer-term consequences of their actions. This explanation uses the same alcohol effects as explanations of alcohol-related accidents in situations requiring alertness and unimpaired cognitive-processing abilities.

(3) Some cultures have defined drinking occasions as situations in which normal restrictions on behaviour do not apply, and drinking and violence are thereby associated. In other words, society defines drinking events as 'time out'. Alcohol intoxication becomes an excuse for excessive and hazardous behaviour, and, generally, behaviour that violates prevailing norms.

(4) Psychological expectancies of alcohol – 'alcohol causes people to behave aggressively' – cause drinkers to behave aggressively. This theory has gained acceptance from psychological experiments using a balanced placebo design: subjects are led to believe that they are drinking alcohol when they are not, and made to think that they are drinking an alcohol-free beverage when they are in fact having a disguised alcoholic drink. Several experiments have shown that the belief that one is drinking alcohol increases strongly the likelihood of aggressive behaviour, which alcohol, at least in low doses, does not. Meta-analyses of these studies, however, indicate that the actual beverage also has an effect at such doses, and that the risk of aggression increases with increasing levels of blood alcohol [99, 100].

DISABILITY AND MORTALITY

Overall, fatal injury is by far the health consequence of alcohol of most concern [101]. Alcohol has been shown, however, to be related more to non-fatal than to fatal outcomes [102, 103]. Worldwide, in 1990 it accounted for 3.5% of the global burden of disease (that is, life years lost owing to premature mortality and to disability together), 1.5% of all deaths, 2.1% of all life years lost, and 6% of all years lost to disability. In other words, alcohol has a much greater impact on disability than on mortality [102].

This ratio is even more pronounced for established market economies such as the European countries, except for the former socialist republics, where 15.6% of all years lost to disability are attributable to alcohol, compared with 5.1% of years lost to premature mortality. It would seem to be more logical in the future, therefore, to concentrate on the non-fatal consequences of alcohol consumption such as disability rather than on mortality. Such a shift would be in line with the overall shift away from mortality as the main indicator of health status [104].

A few recent studies have addressed the association between alcohol consumption and disability. Data from the Swedish Conscript study show that the risk of early disability pension is significantly increased in heavy or 'risky' alcohol consumers [105], whereas Mansson *et al.* [106] found a (bi-variate) J-shaped relationship between alcohol consumption and later disability pension in males. Data on non-mortality outcomes in relation to alcohol consumption are relatively sparse, however, but if the major goal of alcohol epidemiology is better public health then a shift from mortality to disability as outcome in epidemiological studies seems necessary, despite the numerous methodological problems this would entail [107].

SUMMARY AND IMPLICATIONS

Epidemiological studies have demonstrated that alcohol is related to all forms of accident, but the strength of the relationship with categories of accidents varies. The evidence indicates, moreover, that the amount consumed per occasion is the critical feature in determining risk of accidental injury. In workplace accidents, in particular, alcohol apparently plays a certain, but yet minor, role, but this is an area for further scientific study. Although alcohol probably plays a different and more complex role in suicide and attempted suicide than in accidental injury, an extensive research literature shows that it has a significant impact on suicidal behaviour, whether fatal or not. The evidence suggests also that both acute intoxication and chronic abuse increase significantly the risk of intentional self-harm. The relationship between alcohol use and violent behaviour is well established, but countries seem to differ considerably in the strength of this relationship. There is also strong evidence in the literature that social definitions, characteristics of drinking situations and individual predisposing factors, in addition to blood-alcohol concentration, have a determining influence on the risk of violent behaviour in connection with drinking. Recent studies [101, 102] have shown that the relative impact of alcohol on disability is significantly greater than its impact on mortality. Therefore, more attention should be paid to non-mortality effects of alcohol in assessment of the health and social consequences of alcohol consumption.

The epidemiological evidence summarized here indicates that, although heavy drinkers or chronic abusers are at significantly high risk of injury, whether accidental or intentional, it is acute intoxication in the majority of more or less moderate drinkers that is mainly associated with alcohol-related injury. In other words, most of the accidents and injuries in established market economies are caused by usually light to moderate drinkers who were exposed to heavy drinking occasions. Thus, it has been argued that the prevention paradox applies here [108–111], namely that preventive measures to reduce the occurrence of accidents and suicidal behaviour due to alcohol should take the form of population-based strategies aimed at more moderate drinkers, who contribute the most to alcohol-related accidents and intentional injury.

Social consequences

Health consequences such as different forms of physical disability have social repercussions. Depending on the severity of the disability a victim of accident or violence will impose hardships on close relationships. Studies show that most alcohol-related violence occurs between strangers, which would mean that there is little contact between the victim and the person who caused the injury or disability after the event itself. Alcohol-related domestic violence, however, may be considerably underreported, especially in the records of legal authorities.

Fire and traffic accidents can cause facial disfigurement, brain damage and other injuries with serious consequences for social relationships. A French study of adolescents who had been injured in various types of accident requiring at least two days absence from school or being excused from physical-education classes for at least 14 days found that 13% were still troubled by their injury one year later [112]. Musculoskeletal problems predominated, complicating their participation in some sports. Disfiguring scars added to the psychological and social impact of the injury, creating a form a social disability.

The social consequences of suicide and attempted suicide are of several kinds. Firstly, the suffering, loss and guilt that family and friends often experience should be acknowledged. Second, suicidal behaviour has a social 'contagious' effect, particularly among young people, some of whom, shortly afterwards, imitate a suicide or suicide attempt; a single instance of suicidal behaviour may trigger a wave of similar incidents. Thirdly, suicide attempters may be stigmatized, with consequent changed social relationships because their behaviour is considered shameful and unacceptable.

While the health consequences of injuries and fatalities may be interchangeable between the three categories of external trauma, the social consequences will differ according to how an outcome is classified. This is highlighted in cases where the categorization changes with a shift in the attribution of responsibility. A fatal accident in the workplace may be treated as manslaughter or even homicide, with dramatic changes in social consequences. This development re-emerged in some courts in the United States during the 1980s and 1990s, when negligent employers, for instance, received lengthy sentences [113].

Some of the social consequences for the intoxicated person responsible for the trauma may be partly neutralized by the stratagem of defining alcohol-use occasions as at least partly free from the normative strictures of everyday life. Acts committed while intoxicated from alcohol are 'bracketed out'. Individuals who acted in such a way as to cause injury were 'just not their usual selves'. Similar bracketing tactics may be used for behaviour of sober individuals, including 'being under stress', 'not feeling well', 'not being himself', 'having too much to think about' etc. It seems that individuals who have injured or endangered the health of others persist in their belief in such means of bracketing. Those close to the offender accept it as a means of preserving relationships ('when he is sober he is the most gentle man on earth'). Some populations, however, do not permit, in general, the wholesale discounting of responsibility [114]. Despite some difficulties in justifying and adhering strictly to the idea that the intoxicated individual is fully responsible, most countries' laws do not provide for mitigation of a penalty in the case of persons who were intoxicated at the time of an accident or fight. In practice, however, it is easier to divert such persons to treatment, and an intoxicated person accused of homicide is more likely in many countries to be charged with manslaughter than with murder.

It is also true as regards trauma for which an intoxicated person is responsible that at least partial responsibility may be more easily transferred to another, associated person than when a sober individual is responsible. In some court cases in North America, for instance, bar owners have been found guilty because they served a patron an intoxicating amount of alcohol, which later led to an accident or a fight.

The excuse function of alcohol may serve as a bracketing device also for diminishing the stigma of an attempted suicide or an accident, although it may not be generally believed that the individual concerned was not responsible for the incident. Such a device, however, serves no purpose for the victim of an intoxicated car driver or assailant; on the contrary, it can have an aggravating effect. Outrage is often expressed at the mild sentences that courts customarily impose upon drunken drivers who have caused injury or death. The rise of Mothers Against Drunk Driving (MADD) indicates that at least the families of victims of accidents caused by intoxicated people have felt that the social consequences for drunken drivers have not been sufficiently severe.

REFERENCES

1. Roizen, J. (1989) Alcohol and trauma, in *Drinking and Casualties* (eds N. Giesbrecht *et al.*), Tavistock/Routledge, London and New York, pp. 21–66.
2. Österberg, E. (1989) Finnish statistics on alcohol-related accidents, in *Drinking and Casualties* (eds N. Giesbrecht *et al.*), Tavistock/Routledge, London and New York, pp. 215–227.
3. Nordberg, E. (1994) Injuries in Africa – a review. *East African Medical Journal* **71**(6), 339–345.
4. Skog, O.-J. (1989) Trends in alcohol consumption and violent death, in *Drinking and Casualties* (eds N. Giesbrecht *et al.*), Tavistock/Routledge, London and New York, pp. 319–342.
5. Cherpitel, C.J. (1992) Drinking patterns and problems: a comparison of ER patients in an HMO and in the general population. *Alcoholism: Clinical and Experimental Research* **16**, 1104–1109.
6. Hingson, R. and Howland, J. (1987) Alcohol as a risk factor for injury or death resulting from accidental falls: a review of literature. *Journal of Studies on Alcohol* **48**, 212–219.
7. Hingson, R. and Howland, J. (1993) Alcohol and non-traffic unintended injuries. *Addiction* **88**, 877–883.

8. Martin, S.E. (1982) The epidemiology of alcohol-related interpersonal violence. *Alcohol Health and Research World* **16**, 230–237.
9. Martin, S.E. and Bachman, R. (1997) Relationship of alcohol to injury in assault cases, in *Alcohol and Violence* (ed. M. Galanter), Plenum, New York, pp. 41–56 (Vol. 13).
10. Freedland, E.S. et al. (1993) Alcohol and trauma. *Emergency Medicine Clinics of North America* **11**, 225–239.
11. Hurst, P.M. et al. (1994) The Grand Rapids Dip revisited. *Accident Analysis and Prevention* **26**(5), 647–654.
12. United States Department of Health and Human Services. (1997) *Ninth Special Report to the US Congress on Alcohol and Health from the Secretary of Health and Human Services*, US Department of Health and Human Services, Public Health Service, National Institutes of Health, National Institute on Alcohol Abuse and Alcoholism, Washington, (No. 97-4017).
13. Fuller, M.G. (1995) Alcohol use and injury severity in trauma patients. *Journal of Addictive Diseases* **14**, 47–54.
14. Li, G. et al. (1997) Alcohol and injury severity: reappraisal of the continuing controversy. *Journal of Trauma: Injury, Infection, and Critical Care* **42**, 562–569.
15. Wechsler, H. et al. (1969) Alcohol level and home accidents. *Public Health Reports* **84**(12), 1043–1050.
16. Walsh, M.E. and Macleod, D.A.D. (1983) Breath alcohol analysis in the accident and emergency department. *Injury* **15**(1), 62–66.
17. Macdonald, S. et al. (1999) Demographic and substance use factors related to violent and accidental injuries: results from an emergency room study. *Drug and Alcohol Dependence* **55**(1–2), 53–61.
18. Stoduto, G. et al. (1993) Alcohol and drug use among motor vehicle collision victims admitted to a regional trauma unit: demographic, injury, and crash characteristics. *Accident Analysis and Prevention* **25**, 411–420.
19. Lunetta, P. et al. (1998) Water traffic accidents, drowning and alcohol in Finland, 1969–1995. *International Journal of Epidemiology* **27**(6), 1038–1043.
20. Steensberg, J. (1998) Epidemiology of accidental drowning in Denmark 1989–1993. *Accident Analysis and Prevention* **30**(6), 755–762.
21. Barnas, C. et al. (1992) Effects of alcohol and benzodiazepines on the severity of ski accidents. *Acta Psychiatrica Scandinavica* **86**, 296–300.
22. Stinson, F.S. and DeBakey, S.M. (1992) Alcohol-related mortality in the United States, 1979–1988. *British Journal of Addiction* **87**, 777–783.
23. Borkenstein, R.F. et al. (1964) *The Role of the Drinking Driver in Traffic Accidents.* Department of Police Administration, Bloomington, IN.
24. Zador, P.L. (1991) Alcohol-related relative risk of fatal driver injuries in relation to driver age and sex. *Journal of Studies on Alcohol* **52**, 302–310.
25. United States Department of Health and Human Services. (1994) *Eighth Special Report to the US Congress on Alcohol and Health from the Secretary of Health and Human Services*, US Department of Health and Human Services, Public Health Service, National Institutes of Health, National Institute on Alcohol Abuse and Alcoholism, Washington, (No. 94-3699).
26. Single, E. et al. (1998) The economic costs of alcohol, tobacco and illicit drugs in Canada, 1992. *Addiction* **93**(7), 991–1006.
27. Wiebe, J. et al. (1995) Alcohol and drug use in the workplace: a survey of Alberta workers. *American Journal of Health Promotion* **9**, 179–187.
28. Ames, G.M. et al. (1997) The relationship of drinking and hangovers to workplace problems: an empirical study. *Journal of Studies on Alcohol* **58**(1), 37–47.

29. Webb, G.R. et al. (1994) Relationships between high-risk and problem drinking and the occurrence of work injuries and related absences. *Journal of Studies on Alcohol* **55**, 434–446.
30. Gutierrez-Fisac, J.L. et al. (1992) Occupational accidents and alcohol consumption in Spain. *International Journal of Epidemiology* **21**, 1114–1120.
31. Shannon, H.S. et al. (1993) Fatal occupational accidents in Ontario, 1986–1989. *American Journal of Industry Medicine* **23**, 253–264.
32. Hollo, C.D. et al. (1993) Role of alcohol in work-related fatal accidents in Australia 1982–1984. *Occupational Medicine* **43**, 13–17.
33. Naranjo, C.A. and Bremner, K.E. (1993) Behavioural correlates of alcohol intoxication. *Addiction* **88**, 31–41.
34. Sundby, P. (1967) *Alcoholism and Mortality*, Universitetsforlaget, Oslo.
35. Andréasson, S. et al. (1988) Alcohol and mortality among young men:- longitudinal study of Swedish conscripts. *British Medical Journal* **296**, 1021–1025.
36. Rossow, I. and Amundsen, A. (1997) Alcohol abuse and mortality: a 40-year prospective study of Norwegian conscripts. *Social Science and Medicine* **44**, 261–267.
37. Skog, O.-J. (1986) Trends in alcohol consumption and violent deaths. *Brititsh Journal of Addiction* **81**, 365–379.
38. Skog, O.-J. (2001) Alcohol consumption and overall accident mortality in 14 European countries. *Addication* **96**, in press.
39. Cherpitel, C.J. (1995) Alcohol and casualities: comparison of county-wide emergency room data with the county general population. *Addiction* **90**, 343–350.
40. Cherpitel, C.J. (1996) Drinking patterns and problems and drinking in the event: an analysis of injury by cause among casualty patients. *Alcoholism: Clinical and Experimental Research* **20**, 1130–1137.
41. Li, G. et al. (1994) Drinking behavior in relation to cause of death among US adults. *American Journal of Public Health* **84**, 1402–1406.
42. Wells, S. and Macdonald, S. (1999) Relationship between alcohol consumption patterns and car, work, sports and home accidents for different age groups. *Accident Analysis and Prevention* **31**, 663–665.
43. Gruenewald, P.J. and Nephew, T. (1994) Drinking in California: theoretical and empirical analyses of alcohol consumption patterns. *Addiction* **89**, 707–723.
44. Gruenewald, P.J. et al. (1996) Drinking and driving: drinking patterns and drinking problems. *Addiction* **91**, 1637–1649.
45. Treno, A.J. and Holder, H.D. (1997) Measurement of alcohol-involved injury in community prevention: the search for a surrogate III. *Alcoholism: Clinical and Experimental Research* **21**, 1695–1703.
46. Treno, A.J. et al. (1997) Contribution of drinking patterns to the relative risk of injury in six communities: a self-report based probability approach. *Journal of Studies on Alcohol* **58**, 372–381.
47. Cherpitel, C.J. (1996) Regional differences in alcohol and fatal injury: a comparison of data from two county coroners. *Journal of Studies on Alcohol* **57**, 244–248.
48. Moskowitz, H. and Robinson, C. (1988) *Effects of Low Doses of Alcohol on Driving-Related Skills: A Review of the Evidence*, US Department of Transportation, Washington, DC.
49. Krüger, H.P. et al., eds. (1993) *Alcohol, Drugs and Traffic Safety – T'92*. Verlag TÜV Rheinland, Cologne, Germany (Effects of low alcohol dosages: a review of the literature, pp. 763–778).

50. Eckhardt, M.J. et al. (1998) Effects of moderate alcohol consumption on the central nervous system. *Alcoholism: Clinical and Experimental Research* **22**, 998–1040.
51. Nixon, S.J. (1995) Assessing cognitive impairment. *Alcohol Health and Research World* **19**, 97–103.
52. Starmer, G. et al. (1989) Effect of low to moderate doses of alcohol on human performance, in *Human Metabolism of Alcohol*, CRC Press, Boca Raton, pp. 101–130.
53. Mann, R.E. et al. (1998) *Assessing the Potential Impact of Lowering the Legal Blood Alcohol Limit to 50 mg Percent in Canada*, Ontario, Transport Canada, Ottawa.
54. Preusser, D.F. et al. (1978) Driver record evaluation of a drinking driver rehabilitation program. *Journal of Safety Research* **8**, 98–105.
55. Edwards, G. et al. (1994) *Alcohol Policy and the Public Good*, Oxford University Press, Oxford.
56. Lloyd, H.M. and Rogers, P.J. (1997) Mood and cognitive performance improved by a small amount of alcohol given with a lunchtime meal. *Behavioural Pharmacology* **8**, 188–195.
57. Roy, A. and Linnoila, M. (1986) Alcoholism and suicide. *Suicide and Life-Threatening Behavior* **16**, 162–191.
58. Murphy, G.E. and Wetzel, R.D. (1990) The lifetime risk of suicide in alcoholism. *Archives of General Psychiatry* **47**, 383–392.
59. Rossow, I. and Amundsen, A. (1995) Alcohol abuse and suicide: a 40-year prospective study of Norwegian conscripts. *Addiction* **90**, 685–691.
60. Andréasson, S. et al. (1991) Alcohol, social factors and mortality among young men. *British Journal of Addiction* **86**, 877–887.
61. Rossow, I. (1996) Alcohol and suicide – beyond the link at the individual level. *Addiction* **91**(10), 1413–1416.
62. Rygnestad, T. et al. (1992) Fatal and non-fatal repetition of parasuicide, in *Suicidal Behavior in Europe – Recent Research Findings* (eds P. Crepet et al.), London, John Libbey, pp. 183–190.
63. Beck, A.T. et al. (1976) Alcoholism, hopelessness and suicidal behavior. *Journal of Studies on Alcohol* **37**, 66–77.
64. Goodwin, D.W. (1982) Alcoholism and suicide: associated factors, in *The Encyclopedic Handbook in Alcoholism* (eds E.M. Pattison and E. Kaufman), Garner Press, Inc., New York, pp. 655–662.
65. Hawton, K. et al. (1989) Alcoholism, alcohol and attempted suicide. *Alcohol and Alcoholism* **24**, 3–9.
66. Merrill, J. et al. (1992) Alcohol and attempted suicide. *British Journal of Addiction* **87**, 83–89.
67. Salander-Renberg, E. and Jacobsson, L. (1994) Parasuicide in Västerbotten County, Umeå, Sweden 1989–1991, in *Attempted Suicide in Europe – Findings from the Multicentre Study on Parasuicde by the WHO Regional Office for Europe* (eds A.J.F.M. Kerkhof et al.), DSWO Press, Leiden University, Leiden, pp. 87–105.
68. Vega, A.W. et al. (1993) The relationship of drug use to suicide ideation and attempts among African, American, Hispanic, and white non-Hispanic male adolescents. *Suicide and Life-Threatening Behavior* **23**, 110–119.
69. Rossow, I. and Wichtstrøm, L. (1994) Parasuicide and use of intoxicants among Norwegian adolescents. *Suicide and Life-Threatening Behavior* **24**, 174–183.
70. Gruenewald, P.J. et al. (1995) Suicide rates and alcohol consumption in the United States, 1970–89. *Addiction* **90**, 1063–1075.
71. Norström, T. and Rossow, I. (1999) Beverage specific effects on suicide. *Nordic Alcohol and Drug Studies* **16**, 74–82.

72. Hjelmeland, H. (1995) Verbally expressed intentions of parasuicide: I. Characteristics of patients with various intentions. *Crisis* **16**, 176–181.
73. Rossow, I. (1993) Suicide, alcohol and divorce: aspects of gender and family integration. *Addiction* **88**, 1659–1665.
74. Lindberg, S. and Ågren, G. (1988) Mortality among male and female hospitalized alcoholics in Stockholm 1962–1983. *British Journal of Addiction* **83**, 1193–1200.
75. Hasin, D. et al. (1988) Treated and untreated suicide attempts in substance abuse patients. *Journal of Mental and Nervous Disease* **176**, 289–294.
76. Lester, D. (1992) Alcoholism and drug abuse, in *Assessment and Prediction of Suicide* (eds R.W. Maris et al.), Guilford Press, New York, pp. 321–336.
77. Helzer, J.E. and Pryzbeck, T.R. (1988) The co-occurrence of alcoholism with other psychiatric disorders in the general population and its impact on treatment. *Journal of Studies on Alcohol* **49**, 219–224.
78. Norström, T. (1995) Alcohol and suicide: a comparative analysis of France and Sweden. *Addiction* **90**, 1463–1469.
79. Skog, O.-J. et al. (1995) Alcohol and suicide – the Portuguese experience. *Addiction* **90**, 1053–1061.
80. Norström, T. (1988) Alcohol and suicide in Scandinavia. *British Journal of Addiction* **83**, 553–559.
81. Lenke, L. (1990) *Alcohol and Criminal Violence – Time Series Analyses in a Comparative Perspective*, Almqvist and Wiksell, Stockholm.
82. Rossow, I. (2001) Drinking and violence – a cross-cultural comparison of alcohol consumption and homicide rates in 14 European countries. *Addiction* **96**, in press.
83. Shkolnikov, V.M. and Nemtsov, A. (1997) The anti-alcohol campaign and variations in Russian mortality, in *Premature Death in the New Independent States* (eds J.L. Bobadilla et al.), National Academy Press, Washington.
84. Kaasik, T. et al. (1998) The effects of political and economic transitions on health and safety in Estonia: an Estonian-Swedish comparative study. *Social Science and Medicine* **47**, 1589–1599.
85. Shkolnikov, V.M. et al. (1995) Health crisis in Russia. 2. Changes in causes of deaths B comparison with France and England and Wales from 1970 to 1993. *Population* **50**, 945–982.
86. Dahl, E. et al. (1979) Personskader forårsaket av fold. Et 5-årsmateriale av pasienter innlagt i sykehus. *Tidsskrift for Den norske Lægeforening [Journal of the Norwegian Medical Association]* [Injuries caused by violence. A 5-year collection of data on patients admitted to hospital], **30**, 876–879.
87. Melhuus, K. and Sørensen, K. (1997) Vold 1994 – Oslo Legevakt. *Tidsskrift for Den norske Lægeforening [Journal of the Norwegian Medical Association]* [English summary: violence 1994 – Oslo Legevakt], **117**(2), 230–235.
88. Steen, K. and Hunskår, S. Vold i Bergen. (1997) *Tidsskrift for Den norske Lægeforening [Journal of the Norwegian Medical Association]* [English summary: violence in Bergen, Norway], **117**(2), 226–229.
89. Schrøder, H.M. et al. (1992) Epidemiology of violence in a Danish municipality: changes in the incidence during the 1980's. *Danish Medical Bulletin* **39**, 83–83.
90. Pernanen, K. (1991) *Alcohol in Human Violence*, Guilford Press, New York.
91. Goodman, R.A. et al. (1986) Alcohol use and interpersonal violence: alcohol detected in homicide victims. *American Journal of Public Health* **76**, 144–149.
92. Virkkunen, M. (1974) Alcohol as a factor precipitating aggression and conflict behavior leading to homicide. *British Journal of Addiction* **69**, 149–154.
93. Pernanen, K. (1996) *Sammenhengen alkohol-vold* [The Relationship Between Alcohol and Violence], National Institute for Alcohol and Drug Research, Oslo.

94. Roizen, J. (1981) Alcohol and criminal behavior among blacks: the case for research among special populations, in *Drinking and Crime* (eds J.J. Collins), Guilford Press, New York.
95. Brochu, S. *et al.* (2000) Drugs, alcohol and crime: patterns among Canadian federal inmates. *UN Bulletin on Narcotics.*
96. Lillsunde, P. *et al.* (1996) Drugs usage of drivers suspected of driving under the influence of alcohol and/or drugs. A study of one week's samples in 1979 and 1993 in Finland. *Forensic Science International* 77(1–2), 119–129.
97. Rossow, I. (1996) Alcohol-related violence: the impact of drinking pattern and drinking context. *Addiction* 91(11), 1651–1661.
98. Treno, A.J. *et al.* (1998) Sample selection bias in the emergency room: an examination of the role of alcohol in injury. *Addiction* 93(1), 113–129.
99. Hull, J.G. and Bond, C.F. (1986) Social and behavioral consequences of alcohol consumption and expectancy: a meta-analysis. *Psychological Bulletin* 99, 347–360.
100. Bushman, B.J. and Cooper, H.M. (1990) Effects of alcohol on human aggression: an integrative research review. *Psychological Bulletin* 107, 341–354.
101. Single, E. *et al.* (1999) Morbidity and mortality attributable to alcohol, tobacco, and illicit drug use in Canada. *American Journal of Public Health* 89(3), 385–390.
102. Murray, C.J.L. and Lopez, A.D., eds. (1996) *Global Burden of Disease: A Comprehensive Assessment of Mortality and Disability from Diseases, Injuries, and Risk Factors in 1990 and Projected to 2020*, Harvard School of Public Health, Cambridge, MA.
103. Murray, C. and Lopez, A. (1997) Global mortality, disability, and the contribution of risk factors: global burden of disease study. *Lancet* 349, 1436–1442.
104. Beaglehole, R. and Bonita, R. (1997) *Public Health at the Crossroads: Achievements and Prospects*, Cambridge University Press, Cambridge.
105. Upmark, M. *et al.* (1999) Drink driving and criminal behaviours as risk factors for receipt of disability pension and sick leave: a prospective study of young men. *Addiction* 94, 507–519.
106. Mansson, N.O. *et al.* (1999) Alcohol consumption and disability pension among middle-aged men. *Annals of Epidemiology* 9, 341–348.
107. Goerdt, A. *et al.* (1996) Non-fatal health outcomes: concepts, instruments and indicators, in *The Global Burden of Disease: A Comprehensive Assessment of Mortality and Disability from Diseases, Injuries and Risk Factors in 1990 and Projected to 2020* (eds C.J.L. Murray and A.D. Lopez), Harvard School of Public Health, Cambridge, MA, pp. 201–246.
108. Kreitman, N. (1986) Alcohol consumption and the preventive paradox. *British Journal of Addiction* 81, 353–363.
109. Cherpitel, C.J. *et al.* (1995) Alcohol and non-fatal injury in the U.S. general population: a risk function anaylsis. *Accident Analysis and Prevention* 27, 651–661.
110. Norström, T. (1995) Prevention strategies and alcohol policy. *Addiction* 90, 515–524.
111. Skog, O.-J. (1999) The prevention paradox revisited. *Addiction* 94(5), 751–757.
112. Yacoubovitch, J. *et al.* (1995) Sequelae of injuries in adolescents – an epidemiologic study. *Archives de Pédiatrie* 2(6), 532–538.
113. Rosner, D. (2000) When does a worker's death become murder? *American Journal of Public Health* 90(4), 535–540.
114. Paglia, A. and Room, R. (1998) Alcohol and aggression: general population views about causation and responsibility. *Journal of Substance Abuse* 10(2), 199–216.

Chapter eight

Public order and safety

H. Klingemann

The consequences of alcohol use for public order and safety are, like its other social consequences, outcomes of a complex mix of pharmacological effects of alcohol and various social processes. Few if any such consequences for public order and safety will be found in all societies where alcohol is consumed. This is amply borne out in the anthropological literature, which is rich in accounts from pre-industrial societies of the most varied types of post-drinking behaviour. Commonly also in many societies the extent of unruly and dangerous alcohol-related behaviour varies over time. Such geographical, cultural and temporal variations suggested to MacAndrew and Edgerton that all disorderly behaviour after drinking was due to social definitions of drinking events as 'time out', as periods of reprieve from the strictures of everyday sober life, and not to any significant extent to pharmacological effects of alcohol [1].

In Western societies since the temperance days alcohol has been incriminated as a major cause of disorderly (socially disruptive) behaviour and, in its association with crimes of violence, the most serious threat to order and safety [2]. Violent crime is only an extreme case, however. Analytically, socially disruptive effects of alcohol may be placed on a *continuum* of deviant behaviour, involving all forms of deviance, nuisance and threat to safety and the social and physical environment, such as 'contribution of alcohol consumption to noise', 'loss of sleep of neighbours of bars', 'harassment in the streets and parks' and 'littering of beer cans in tourist centres'.

By deviating from behaviour that is socially approved, disorderly and dangerous behaviour triggers responses from the formal and informal agents of social control – the police, the employer, the welfare worker, the reference group or the public in general. To measure and count social consequences in this domain, it is useful to take as starting points the different social agents and

Harald Klingemann and Gerhard Gmel (eds.), *Mapping the Social Consequences of Alcohol Consumption*, 113–132.
© 2001 *Kluwer Academic Publishers. Printed in Great Britain.*

sources of public reaction. Informal and formal social reactions vary, of course, from one country, culture and social context to another. The cultural context and its limits of tolerance partly determine what constitutes violation of public order and its attribution to alcohol abuse. The cultural context is useful also for disentangling the indirect effects and costs of social control from the direct effects of the behaviour attributed to alcohol abuse.

Alcohol acts in several separate ways: in the event, in setting the stage for events, in attracting individuals to high-risk social contexts and situations, and in other ways. It acts pharmacologically in creating public disorder and endangering safety, but it also raises issues by its symbolic significance and visibility and by the reactions it elicits from authorities and the public.

THE ROLE OF ALCOHOL IN CRIME: POLICE AND THE CRIMINAL JUSTICE SYSTEM AS GUARDIANS OF 'THE PUBLIC ORDER'

Without question alcohol plays a major role in crime, especially crimes of violence. Rates of violent crime are directly related to level of alcohol consumption: as consumption increases in a society, so too does the rate of violent crime. Norström [3] calculated that changes in total alcohol consumption in Sweden between 1956 and 1994 accounted for 47% of the changes in the country's assault rate, and as much as 68% of the homicide rate. Countries vary greatly, however, in the closeness of this relationship between total consumption and crime, which indicates that drinking patterns and social factors not directly related to level of consumption also play a part.

The category of assaults and homicide incidents is that with the highest level of alcohol involvement, though countries vary widely in this regard. This variation makes it difficult to determine the proportions of assaults and homicides in which either the perpetrator or the victim, or both, had been drinking. The following ranges are based on soundly designed and conducted studies with relatively large samples: Sweden 75–85%, Norway 70–80%, Finland 65–75%, USA 55–65%, and Canada 35–45%. Part of the apparent inter-country variation may be attributable to differences in the perception of alcohol as a causal factor in violent crime and the associated care with which the police or other authorities record its presence. The degree to which alcohol is involved in rape or robbery has not been studied to the same extent, and studies vary widely in their findings as to whether those who committed such crimes were drinking at the time. For different violent crimes, studies have reported ranges of from 13% for sex offences to 87% for homicide [4, p. 9].

The law in Western countries does not, in general, specify intoxication as an extenuating factor, but if the perpetrator, and especially if the victim also, was under the influence of alcohol the courts in many countries are more likely to treat homicide as manslaughter than as murder [5]. Survey research also shows that the general public in many countries does not consider drunkenness a valid excuse for violent behaviour, or that intoxicated individuals have diminished responsibility for their actions [6].

Intoxicated individuals are easy prey for robbers and thieves. Moore and Gerstein suggest that '[T]he least arguable connection between alcohol and crime is that drunks are easy and traditional prey for criminal harm' [7, p. 106]. City-planning factors can interact with the incapacitation of the drunken person, as when public drinking places and public drunkenness are concentrated in particular areas. Victims of homicide often have significantly higher blood-alcohol levels than common levels for impaired driving in European countries [8, 9].

The direct social consequences of alcohol-related deviant behaviour for the individual and partner or family members, such as imprisonment, treatment, or stigmatization, will differ according to how the courts treat such behaviour and the public views it. The direct costs are relatively easy to survey. In the United States for 1992 they were calculated at US$ 6712 million for criminal justice expenditure and health care of victims. Estimated crime-related productivity losses from alcohol in the same year were US$ 13 050 million.

Alcohol abuse also has a more long-term effect in that it leads to conflict with those in a position to designate an individual's behaviour as disorderly, unsafe or deviant and to penalize such behaviour. In the most serious cases the penalties may have the effect of placing problem drinkers in environments that put them at high risk of more serious social disorder.

COMPULSORY TREATMENT AND 'DANGER TO THE PUBLIC': TREATMENT AND CRIMINAL JUSTICE COOPERATING IN THE INTERESTS OF THE PUBLIC ORDER

The relationship between alcohol and disturbance of the public order is partly reflected in regulations that provide for compulsory civil committal and treatment under compulsion from the criminal justice system. As a comparative study of legislation carried out for the World Health Organization has shown, the mental-health legislation of many countries specifies 'dangerous behaviour' resulting from drug or alcohol dependence as grounds for committal to an institution. The legislative wording differs to some extent, but the rationale of committal is threats to public safety and public order: 'danger to public safety' (Germany); 'seriously and repeated disturbance of the public order' (Hungary); 'serious danger to the life or health of others' (Norway); 'violation of the public order or the rules of socialist community life' (USSR); 'disorderly behavior' (USA) [13, pp. 45, 50–53]. How these general clauses are applied in practice may be illustrated by the case of Sweden:

> Under Swedish legislation on the detention of intoxicated persons, any person found in a public place in a state of intoxication, caused by

> Costs of alcohol abuse for specific and related crime, 1992 (billion $) [10]:
> - Criminal justice expenditure and health care of victim: US$ 6.712
> - Crime-related productivity losses: US$ 13.050
>
> Economic costs of alcohol misuse and alcoholism in the United States, 1975 (billion $)
> - Violent crime: 2.86
> - Social responses: 1.94 [11, p. 207]
>
> Empirical studies on alcohol use and rape (police reports):
> - Alcohol offenders (4 studies): 13–37%; alcohol victims: 6–36%. [12, p. 19]
>
> Evidence of intoxication at time of homicide
> - Victims (29 studies): 14–87%
> - Offenders (3 studies): 24–37% [12, p. 9]
>
> Effects of total alcohol consumption (Sweden 1956–1994) on:
> - Assault rate: 47% attributable fraction
> - Homicide rate: 68% attributable fraction [3, pp. 693, 695].

alcoholic beverages or other intoxicants, may be detained by a policeman if his condition renders him unable to look after himself or he is otherwise dangerous to himself or others. The police are required to assist such persons in seeking medical and social aid and assistance [13, p. 48].

Compulsory confinement in a treatment institution, or involuntary treatment, is used as a legal response to alcohol-related social behaviour considered to be deviant but not severe enough to warrant intervention by the criminal justice system. In this way, as long as a causal link with substance use can be established, the control of public disorder or danger is provided for by placing it under the umbrella of 'treatment'. In his review of studies of compulsory treatment for non-drink-driving offenders, Polcin [14, p. 139] points out that such arrests are common among the homeless, welfare recipients, low-income individuals, the poorly educated, and single males. On the basis of this clustering, one might conclude that statistics on compulsory treatment could serve as an indication of the occurrence of a range of alcohol-related social problems such as public drinking, violence in the private sphere, fights and quarrels. The percentage of patients involuntarily committed, however, has decreased in many countries since the 1960s and reached a minimum level in the 1970s (for Finland see [15, p. 93], for Sweden see [16, p. 74], for Austria see [17, p. 102]), indicating that international trends, such as the movement towards decarceration, overshadow factual changes in alcohol-related problems. Figure 1 shows the decline in involuntary admissions as a proportion of total admissions for Switzerland.

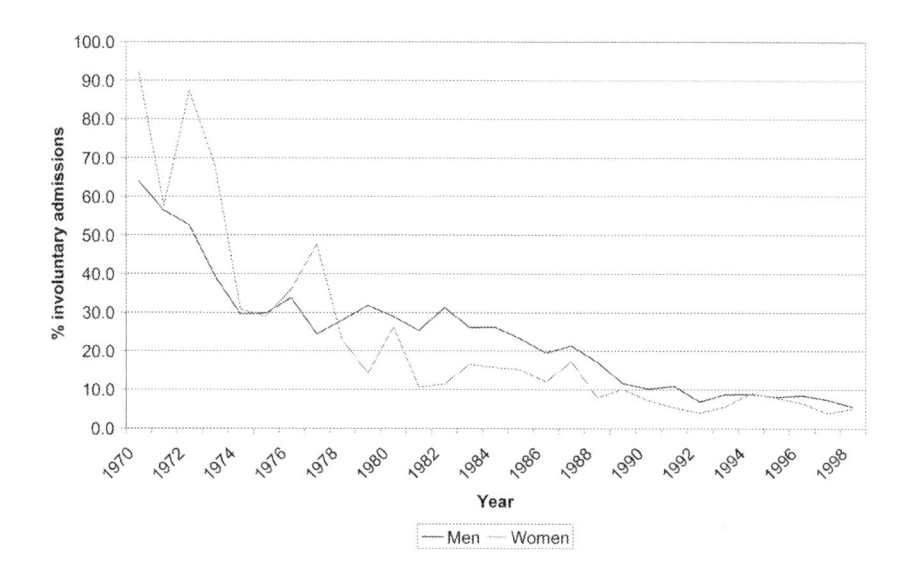

Figure 1 Alcohol clinics in Switzerland: involuntary admissions as a proportion of total admissions, 1970–1998. [Source: [18] 1970–1981; SAKRAM statistics – SIPA (own calculations) 1982–1998].

THE IMPACT OF ALCOHOL CONSUMPTION ON THE PHYSICAL AND SOCIAL ENVIRONMENT, AND COMMUNAL/MUNICIPAL AUTHORITIES AS REPRESENTATIVES OF THE PUBLIC ORDER

Municipalities often have to deal with, and regulate, negative social consequences of alcohol consumption in their communities and, at the same time, take account of political interests (see [19] for a historical example). Premises licensed to sell alcohol disturb neighbourhoods. Noise from bars, public houses and hotels with late closing or lively 'happy hours' constitutes a public nuisance. Litter as cans or glass bottles is a nuisance and a safety risk. Women are victimized in and outside bars [20]. Fear of crime, vandalism and graffiti diminish property values and cause concern about the preservation of a distinctive atmosphere and the reputation of a town as a clean and orderly tourist attraction [21, p. 45]. A number of studies using police or emergency-room data and participant observation have found high rates of violent incidents involving alcohol in licensed premises [22, 23]. Misdirected attempts to control aggression can aggravate the problem, however. Wells *et al.* show in their overview that a permissive attitude towards the behaviour of patrons, and the intervention of security staff, often *initiated* violent behaviour [24, p. 818]. Against this should be weighed the *benefits* from neighbourhood drinking places in the form of socializing, as a way to increase the attractiveness of an area as a lively quarter, and a possible fall in rates of other forms of crime when a certain amount of informal social control is being exerted late into the night.

> Evidence suggests that a large proportion of violent crime occurs in and around licensed premises [24, p. 818].
>
> In Australia 40% of alcohol-related accidents stem from drinking in licensed establishments [25]

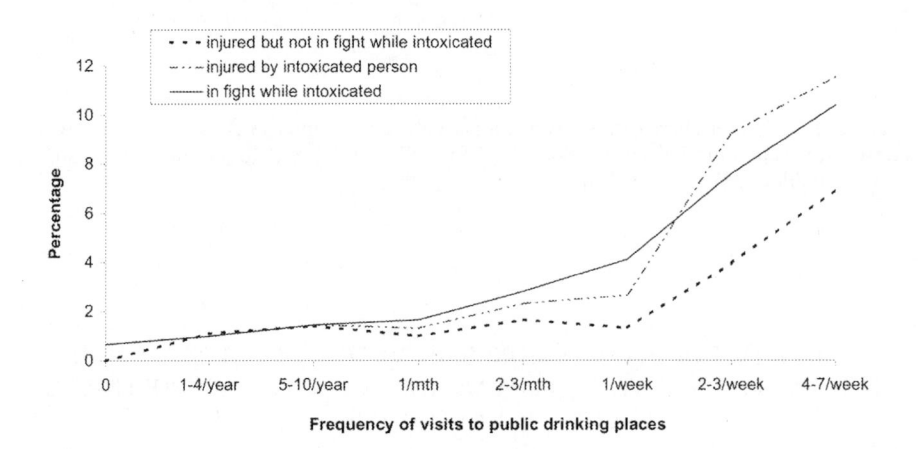

Figure 2 Percentage of respondents who reported taking part in a fight while intoxicated, being injured by an intoxicated person, and being injured from other causes, in the past 12 months, as related to frequency of visits to public drinking places during the same period. [Source: 27, p. 1656].

Conflicting interests and perceived social consequences become visible in communal zoning and land-use changes which would affect residents and properties in the neighbourhoods (see e.g. Phipps' [26] analysis of decisions of the Liquor License Board of Ontario regarding a liquor licence for a night club). The extensive literature on community prevention provides a broader framework for this response of communal authorities.

ALCOHOL CONSUMPTION AS PART OF DEVIANT LIFE-STYLES? SKID ROWS AND THE HOMELESS: WELFARE AGENCIES, SOCIAL WORK AND NEIGHBOURHOODS WITH VESTED INTERESTS IN PUBLIC ORDER

Social consequences of alcohol abuse include loss of work and estrangement from partners and friends (see Chapters 5, 6 and 7 of this volume), which may lead eventually to complete exclusion or withdrawal from the conventional social world. Welfare agencies and social workers, and to a lesser extent the criminal justice system, subject skid-row areas, individual street drinkers, open alcohol (and drug) scenes, and the homeless to a mix of care and control (for a more extensive discussion see [28]). The loss of 'normal' social networks and the rigours of life on the street are generally considered to be negative social consequences, in many cases at least partly attributable to alcohol consumption. Some homeless people, however, seek and appreciate this 'life-style' as a means of increasing satisfaction with life. Rubington in his classic work on chronic drunkenness offenders on Skid Row underlines the *positive functions* of this subculture: 'Social support, which the respectable world withdraws, comes from one's associates on Skid Row with less effort. Existence within the Skid-Row community of internal negative reference groups makes it possible for some even to deny the facts of status fall' [29, p. 148].

Today's 'zero tolerance' policies applied to crime, drugs and vagrancy have been justified by the assumption that intervention at an early stage of deviance and its outward signs (such as broken windows in a neighbourhood) will eventually deter people from committing more serious criminal acts and ultimately strengthen conformity: 'Order maintenance policing involves the use of law enforcement resources to attack visible signs of disorder ... [P]ublic drunkenness, prostitution, aggressive panhandling and similar behaviour signal that the community is unable or unwilling to enforce basic norms of civility' [30, pp. 823, 882]. Along similar lines, Herring describes policy landmarks in England, where in the 1980s the perceived public nuisance and 'anti-social behaviour' of street drinkers and 'abusive winos' in town centres attracted attention and local authorities introduced bans and by-laws making it an offence to consume 'intoxicating liquor in a designated place upon being warned by a constable not to do so' [31, p. 188]. This policy leaves much to the discretion of the police officer, while civil rights may remain unprotected and hidden political agendas may be pursued. Such repressive measures may result, therefore, in such negative social consequences as the de facto criminalization of alcoholism and homelessness. This is reflected in United States survey data showing that 'within welfare agencies 51% of the individuals with alcohol abuse problems had contact with the criminal justice system within the past year alone' [14, p. 139]. The costs and benefits of social work and treatment interventions ('outreach' and 'intensive case management') as social-control consequences are difficult to assess [32, 33].

> (USA survey data) 'Within welfare agencies 51% of the individuals with alcohol abuse problems had contact with the criminal justice system within the past year alone' [14, p. 139]

DRINKING AND OCCUPATIONAL CAREERS: CONFLICTS AT THE WORKSITE AND DISCRIMINATION IN THE LABOUR MARKET

Clinical studies of alcohol abusers illustrate the damage which alcohol consumption inflicts upon the social networks of drinkers in their private relations or in secondary groups, disturbing work relations and career opportunities [11, p. 216]. Early onset of alcohol abuse significantly retards educational attainment [34]. For young people in general, heavy drinking can curtail their education and stifle job opportunities [35].

The misuse of alcohol results in substantial economic costs or loss of labour-market productivity [36], in part through direct health consequences of alcohol use, such as physical injuries in the workplace, and from absenteeism. The specifically *social* consequences of alcohol consumption for 'order in the workplace' and resulting conflict are reflected in the efforts of employers to control the problem by implementing drug-alcohol testing schemes or Employee Assistance Programmes [37], and to neutralize workplace subcultures in which heavy drinking is not only accepted but also encouraged (see [38, 39] on occupational subcultures with norms that promote drinking in a hospital environment). More precisely, Ames *et al.* [40] have shown a significant relationship between hangover and numerous workplace problems such as 'falling asleep', 'having had an argument or fight' and 'having argued with the supervisor'. Richman *et al.* [41] point out that sexual harassment and general workplace harassment are among other social occurrences significantly linked with alcohol abuse and other drug use.

The causal link between alcohol abuse and unemployment is complex: problem drinking may reduce employment [36, p. 432] but unemployment also *increases* alcohol use and abuse [42].

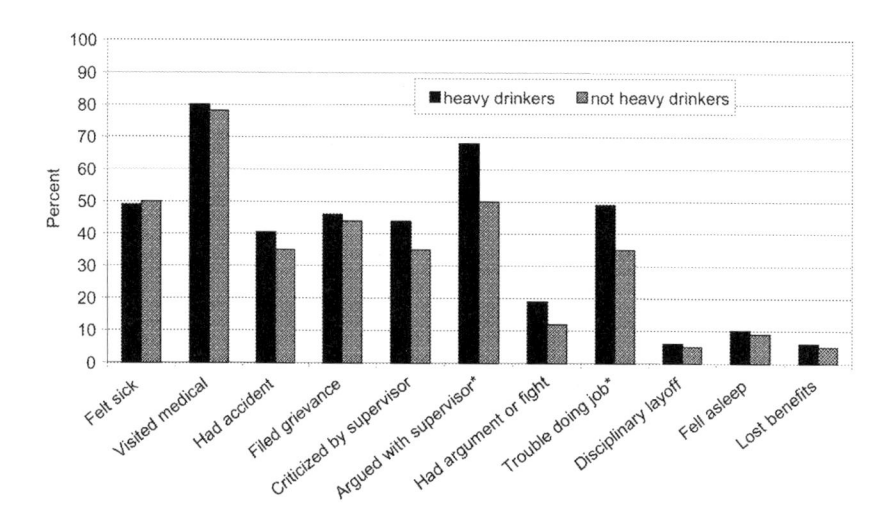

Figure 3 Relationships between heavy drinking and workplace problems (*$p<0.05$). [Source: 40].

In older age-groups alcohol abuse and workloads may become increasingly incompatible and lead to 'role shrinkage' or 'disengagement' from social networks, reduced work performance and possibly early retirement [35]. Job loss and forced retirement can be assumed to have serious consequences for the individual's social status, prestige and wellbeing.

PUBLIC ORDER AND CULTURAL ASPECTS: SOCIAL CLIMATE AND LEVEL OF TOLERANCE

A group of Dutch researchers defines 'social climate on alcohol' as 'the blend of different views on drinking, conceptions of alcohol-related problems, and the defining of appropriate measures for dealing with them' [45, p. 141]. This blend of views is not uniform; while some alcohol-related views may develop in a liberal direction, others may become less permissive. Polarization of opinion regarding the control of physical, demographic or economic access to alcohol may well co-exist with lack of polarization on whether drunken customers should be served or on the provision of information about treatment.

In a cross-cultural perspective Gerstein noted that 'arrest rates for public drunkenness vary slightly inversely with total consumption of alcohol ... the

> Trends in % of workers aged 18–49 reporting heavy use of alcohol [43, pp. 9, 11]
>
> | 1985 | 1988 | 1990 | 1991 | 1992 | 1993 |
> |------|------|------|------|------|------|
> | 8.5% | 6.5% | 6.8% | 7.6% | 7.0% | 7.0% |
>
> Construction workers:
>
> | | | 19% | 16% | 18% | 12% | 13% |
> |---|---|-----|-----|-----|-----|-----|
>
> National Health Interview Survey (1988; $n=35\,000$) results:
>
> After eliminating potential bias due to reverse causality, evidence was found that non-employment significantly reduces both alcohol consumption and dependence syndromes ... involuntary unemployment had a mixed effect, job loss increased the consumption of alcohol in the overall sample but reduced dependence symptoms among single respondents [44]

wetter the country the less concerned its citizens are to see their drunken fellows whisked into police vans' [11, p. 216].

In his overview of the WHO project on public drinking, Eric Single points out that countries and cultures differ considerably in their perception of social problems. It is of interest that countries with tolerant attitudes towards public drunkenness had the most arrests for public drunkenness while, conversely, the intolerant had the fewest; Single concludes that '... social norms accepting or disapproving of drunken comportment have a greater impact on behavior than on legislation' [46, p. 437]. As we have seen above, it is not only perceptions that vary: Lenke [47] found that the relationship between per capita alcohol consumption and criminal violence varied with cultural context. The link between level of consumption and violence is weak in France and relatively strong in the 'dry' cultures of the Nordic countries of Finland, Norway and Sweden [3, see also Chapter 7].

Regional differences in the societal climate within the same country may also be expressed in higher or lower tolerance of alcohol-related disturbances of the public order. An interesting case study in this connection relates to noise from Bavarian beer gardens. On an application by neighbours of a beer garden, a local court imposed a closing time of 9.30 p.m. This led to the 'First Beer Garden Revolution', in 1995, when 20 000 people demonstrated in the streets of Munich against the early closing hour. The State of Bavaria then issued regulations permitting a one-hour extension. On appeal, a federal court ruled that the State regulations had legal flaws and were not compatible with federal law on noise protection, as they did not define noise limits precisely but referred rather to the 'traditional high acceptance of noise from beer gardens'. An additional shortcoming was that the Bavarian authorities had not found it necessary to define what premises qualified as beer gardens, 'because every child in Bavaria knows what a beer garden is'. A second State regulation with more clearly defined rules came into effect in May 1999. During this 'campaign' local feelings ran high: 'the beer gardens will not be sacrificed on the altar of the central state' and 'the culture and tradition of the state needs to be protected' were slogans representing the 'Free State' of Bavaria as pitted against 'Prussian' rulings from Berlin; organizers stopped short of getting under way a protest march to Berlin with 1000 tractors [48].

It can be concluded that the perception of alcohol-related noise as a threat to health [49] is culturally variable, even within countries. In Norway, the Oslo authorities have had to grapple with the social consequences of licensed establishments, imposing various local opening hours throughout the 1990s. Public drinking places more than doubled in number during this period [50] and the authorities made successive attempts to find a balance that would satisfy the various interest groups such as the police, the bar owners, the temperance movement, the tourist industry, and various segments of the general public.

In other countries, as the social climate regarding alcohol changes over time, perceptions of alcohol-related social harm change accordingly. In the Netherlands, for instance, changes that were evident in such specific regards as tolerance towards drinking behaviour of close relatives and drinking behaviour at parties (which increased considerably between 1958 and 1994 [45, p. 147]), were reflected in attitudes towards issues of public order and towards the authorities in particular.

These results indicate that perception of social harm and benefits from alcohol consumption will depend on the societal definitions and the climate of public opinion in each country. Alcohol consumption as a social issue may lead to widespread conflict between social groups, as described in the Bavarian case study, but it can also increase cohesion in society, and lead to the mobilization of grass-roots movements and lay-help in general, as the example of Mothers Against Drunk Driving (MADD) shows [51, 52]. Such social consequences cannot be explained without taking into account, in addition to public views on alcohol use and the perceptions of a great number, social phenomena sometimes far removed from the direct consequences of drinking. Alcohol is integrated with the social life of societies, and the issues that determine social consequences of alcohol are not limited to the beverage itself.

Social climate on alcohol:

United States and Canada: (1989–90]: There was greater polarization of opinion within each country regarding policy items relating to promotion of alcohol or control of physical, demographic or economic access than with regard to curtailing service to drunken customers or providing information about treatment [53].

Netherlands [45, p. 144] (1980/81 vs.1994), *against* ...

Prohibition of advertising	52%	vs.	41%
Price increase	42%	vs.	32%
Restriction of alcohol use in public places	78%	vs.	81%
Raising age limits	62%	vs.	62%
Reduction of public houses	30%	vs.	29%
Reduction of shops selling alcohol	33%	vs.	33%

SYMBOLIC PUBLIC DISPLAY AND POTENTIAL OFFENCE TO ONLOOKERS OF ALCOHOL AS A COMMODITY: MORAL CRUSADERS DEFENDING THE PUBLIC ORDER OR CONTROLLING THE POOR?

Especially in North America and the Nordic countries public drunkenness and drinking in public, as well as the open display of alcohol, have been considered to imply negative social consequences. Such behaviour is at least partly controlled when confined to relatively closed settings such as bars or public houses or stadiums. In open public areas such as streets or parks it produces the same kinds of harm, possibly only worse (unmuffled noise, indiscriminate littering, etc). The visibility and the potential for bad modelling undermine public values and morals, and represent a symbolic affront to values held by large segments of society (on modelling delinquent behaviour see [54]). 'Brown bagging' in the American South – bringing one's own alcohol in a brown bag to an unlicensed pub – is an historical instance of ways to hinder unwanted public displays. The Canadian regulation requiring public drinking places to conceal the bar scene from the street by curtains is another. Many regulations are not about the potential situational risk of alcohol (cf. firearms) but about symbolic displays and potential offence to onlookers. The regulations in the United States against open containers of alcohol are often used to restrict the behaviour of teenagers in public places – groups of teenagers holding open cans or bottles are often regarded as menacing.

Since 1970 the trend in the United States and in most other countries has been to decriminalize public drunkenness [11, p. 218, 46, p. 436]. From a recent assessment in the United States, however, it appears that local ordinances, and often state laws, against drinking in public are not relics of Prohibition but, rather, recently adopted provisions. Limitations have gradually been imposed upon freedom to behave in a self-destructive or deviant way in public, as exemplified by smoking regulations in public buildings such as banks, administration offices, airports and train stations.

Alcohol regulations can be used as a pretext to control deviant behaviour in a grey zone where the treatment or criminal justice system cannot intervene, or simply as part of a hidden political agenda. Historically, the 'pub' as the meeting place for working-class people was to some extent also a political arena. At the time, one would have classified the 'destabilization of the political order' by drinking together in public places as a social consequence or cost of alcohol. A modern parallel would be the use of alcohol regulations to control the lifestyle of youth or of youth subcultures.

Recent developments in the USA: 'Local ordinances and often state laws against drinking in public have been quite recently adopted in many places in the US. Also laws against having an open alcohol container in an automobile. Alcohol regulations are not about the potential in-the-moment danger of the commodity (as with firearms) but about symbolic displays and potential offense to an onlooker. The regulations against open alcohol containers are often used to restrict the behaviour of teenagers in public places – groups of teenagers with open cans or bottles in their hands are often viewed as potentially menacing.

Every American state has a thick volume of the 'alcoholic beverage control laws', and there are often county and municipal regulations on top of these. The degree of enforcement of their different aspects varies, but has probably been increasing as alcohol becomes more contested territory again in the US in recent years' [55]

DRINKING AND ALCOHOL IN YOUTH SUBCULTURES: YOUTH AND ALCOHOL IN CONFLICT WITH THE DOMINANT CULTURE (CONTROLLING YOUTH)

The prominent role of alcohol at colleges and universities (drinking games, rites of initiation) has become – especially in the United States – a matter of concern to university authorities, parents and student bodies. The social tissue and achievement orientation in this area has been harmed by this kind of 'drinking sport'. Fatal accidents and alcohol poisoning have occurred, and such drinking patterns have been known to set vulnerable students up for a deviant career. Wechsler *et al.* [56] report that binge drinkers among American college students in *both* 1993 and 1997 were at increased risk of alcohol-related problems, and non-bingers at colleges with high rates of binge-drinking were at increased risk of encountering indirect effects of binge drinking, ranging from common annoyance to vandalism and assault.

The function which problem drinking plays as a gateway to juvenile crime, including minor offences such as property damage (graffiti), theft and assault, needs to be more closely analysed. Recent research has focused on the symbolic significance of drinking in defining lifestyles and identities of young people. Drinking behaviour is related to the wider social transition towards adulthood [57]. The social consequences and, in particular, the symbolic *positive* significance of drinking patterns in various phases of lifetime change need to be considered in order to achieve a balanced assessment.

HOOLIGANISM – 'EPISODIC' ANTISOCIAL, DELINQUENT BEHAVIOUR: SOCIAL WORKERS, POLITICIANS AND THE PUBLIC AS GUARDIANS OF 'THE PUBLIC ORDER'

Alcohol consumption seems to trigger outbreaks of violence at sports events (e.g. soccer matches) and is often correlated with group-type crimes of a racist or ideological nature [58]. Examples are the numerous acts of violence committed by soccer fans during the 1998 World Cup competition in France (Alcohol Alert 1998), including the attempt by four German soccer fans ('The Hamburg Ultras') to murder a French policeman; they later entered a plea of 'not guilty' on the grounds of extreme intoxication. Verleyen and Smet found that 35% of the hooligans they studied were out of work, had a lower social-class background and were addicted to alcohol and drugs [59]. Conversely, van Limbergen, Colaers and Walgrave [60, p. 7], who analysed 306 football games in the Belgian 1986–1987 season, claim: 'There was no, or only a weak relation with factors that are sometimes mentioned in relationship to hooliganism: sale of alcohol, the importance of the match, the result of the match, the time of the match (afternoon or evening) and so on'. They stress that football hooligans who attach themselves to a club are attracted to the subcultural 'near group' because of their social vulnerability.

Skinheads and groups motivated by fascist ideas and who engage in the 'bashing' of foreigners, gays and 'leftists' often act under the influence of alcohol. Members of these groups are often fully integrated into society but 'come out' during leisure time or weekends. This alcohol-related network has considerable impact on the fear of crime, the wellbeing of citizens, and the network of tolerance in society, and this impact needs to be measured in local surveys of public perceptions.

> Hooliganism – how can the European Union stamp it out?
>
> 'Increased and free movement of people has sadly aided the hooligans who prey on major sporting events. The European Union is active in seeking to put a stop to hooliganism. It has put in place a joint strategy, including the exchange between different countries of information on known trouble-makers, the joint assessment of risks involved in international fixtures, shared details of travel arrangements to away matches, and a network of liaison officers to combat hooliganism. Measures for a coordinated European Union approach to ticket sales, drinking at sports events, and the design and safety of sports areas are also being examined at European level'.[1]

CONCLUDING REMARKS: IMPLICATIONS FOR POLICY-MAKERS

In Western societies, since the time of the temperance movement, alcohol has been considered a major cause of deviant behaviour, ranging from disorderly, socially disruptive conduct to serious threats to order and safety. This is widely recognised on the part of the general public, the police and criminal justice system, health authorities and medical care providers, communal authorities, welfare agencies and employers. All realise, for this reason, that alcohol consumption needs to be controlled. To some extent, the cultural context and its limits of tolerance partly determine what constitutes violation of public order and how much is attributable to alcohol abuse, but it is clear from a large body of research evidence that the threats that alcohol presents for public order and safety are actual, not merely socially or culturally perceived, constructed or defined.

Specific findings

- Without question, alcohol plays a major role in crime, especially crimes of violence. With some variation in international comparison, the category of assaults and homicides is that with the highest level of alcohol involvement, ranging between 35% (Canada) and 85% (Sweden).
- Clinical studies of alcohol abusers illustrate the damage which alcohol consumption inflicts upon working relationships and career opportu-

---

[1] European Commission Fact sheets/ www.cec.org.uk/pubs/facts/culture/chap3.htm

nities. Numerous workplace problems, including sexual and other forms of harassment, are linked with the use of alcohol and other drugs.

- A tolerant social climate toward public drunkenness goes together with high arrest rates, and vice versa, which suggests that informal social control has a greater influence on behaviour than legislation. Both are necessary, however, to reach an optimum of costs, control and acceptable public order.

- Alcohol or alcohol abuse often triggers highly visible disruptive behaviour such as football hooliganism and racial violence or is used as an excuse to deny responsibility or advanced as a mitigating factor to escape punishment.

As this overview has shown, we witness to some extent an *increased* sensitivity to the social consequences and costs of so-called 'antisocial' behaviour in general (not in the clinical sense). This in turn leads to a less accurate and wider interpretation by the authorities of the concept of '*alcohol*-induced problems and disturbance of the public order'.

Alcohol control measures used to increase public safety and order should be based on evidence rather than morality. Policy measures designed to control 'difficult' or disadvantaged groups (e.g. youth subcultures, the poor and the homeless) by reducing broad socio-political issues to an alcohol-only issue are counterproductive to an efficient alcohol policy with high credibility, in the long run. Civil rights have to be respected, especially in implementing so-called 'zero tolerance policies'. Punitive or control measures must not add to cultural or social stigma or have the effect of exposing drinkers to environments that conduce to even more serious social disorder.

Involuntary committal of alcohol abusers to inpatient psychiatric facilities constitutes a major interference with their lives; such committals should be exclusively for purposes of treatment, not for reasons of convenience of families or partners or of threats to their safety, which should be dealt with in other ways. Involuntary committals, however, have decreased in many countries since the 1960s, probably because the use of the 'umbrella of alcohol treatment' to control public disorder or danger has been seen to be an unwarranted or ineffective course of action.

Liberalization and deregulation in relation to outlet density and opening hours will induce an increase in alcohol-related disturbances to public order and threats to safety, the costs and the burden of which the taxpayer and the general public have to shoulder. Evidence indicates that a large proportion of violent crime occurs in and around licensed premises. Outbreaks of violence associated with mass sports events and other cultural events may be avoided if such events are required to be alcohol-free.

Measures to increase public awareness of alcohol problems should highlight the threat that alcohol poses to safety and public order. More such problems are likely to come to attention at first, but the public may then demand and support countermeasures. For example, the vulnerability of intoxicated individuals to criminal harm may be used as a starting point for community planners. Public attention to this matter may bring about protective measures such as social support and skilled help to individuals or families rendered vulnerable by alcoholism.

ACKNOWLEDGEMENTS

Special thanks go to Kai Pernanen for his critical reading of the initial manuscript and selected additions.

REFERENCES

1. MacAndrew, C. and Edgerton, R.B. (1969) *Drunken Comportment*. Aldine, Chicago.
2. Fahrenkrug, H.W. (1984) *Alkohol, Individuum und Gesellschaft. Zur Sozialgeschichte des Alkoholproblems in den USA*, Campus Verlag, Frankfurt.
3. Norström, T. (1998) Effects on criminal violence of different beverage types and private and public drinking. *Addiction* 93(5), 689–699.
4. Roizen, J. (1997) Epidemiological issues in alcohol-related violence, in *Recent Developments in Alcoholism* (ed. M. Galanter), Plenum Press, New York/London, pp. 7–37.
5. Fischer, B. and Rehm, J. (1998) Intoxication, the law and criminal responsibility – A sparkling cocktail at times: the case studies of Canada and Germany. *European Addiction Research* 4(3), 89–101.
6. Paglia, A. and Room, R. (1998) Alcohol and aggression: general population views about causation and responsibility. *Journal of Substance Abuse* 10(2), 199–216.
7. Moore, M.H. and Gerstein, D.R. (1981) *Alcohol and Public Policy: Beyond the Shadow of Prohibition*, National Academy Press, Washington, DC.
8. Virkkunen, M. (1974) Alcohol as a factor precipitating aggression and conflict behavior leading to homicide. *British Journal of Addiction* 69, 149–154.
9. Goodman, R.A. *et al.* (1986) Alcohol use and interpersonal violence: alcohol detected in homicide victims. *American Journal of Public Health* 76, 144–149.
10. Harwood, H.J. *et al.* (1999) Cost estimates for alcohol and drug abuse. *Addiction* 94(5), 631–635.
11. Gerstein, D.R. (1981) Alcohol use and consequences, in *Alcohol and Public Policy: Beyond the Shadow of Prohibition* (eds M.H. Moore and D.R. Gerstein), National Academy Press, Washington, DC, pp. 182–224.
12. Fuller, R.K. (1997) Overview, in *Recent Developments in Alcoholism* (ed. M. Galanter), Plenum Press, New York/London, pp. 3–5.
13. Porter, L. *et al.* (1986) *The Law and the Treatment of Drug- and Alcohol-Dependent Persons*, World Health Organization, Geneva.
14. Polcin, D.L. (1999) Criminal justice coercion in the treatment of alcohol problems: an examination of two client subgroups. *Journal of Psychoactive Drugs* 31(2), 137–143.

15. Takala, J.-P. and Lehto, J. (1992) The non-medical model reconsidered, in *Cure, Care, or Control – Alcoholism Treatment in Sixteen Countries* (eds H. Klingemann *et al.*), State University of New York Press, Albany, pp. 87–110.
16. Rosenqvist, P. and Kurube, N. (1992) Dissolving the Swedish alcohol-treatment system, in *Cure, Care, or Control – Alcoholism Treatment in Sixteen Countries* (eds H. Klingemann *et al.*), State University of New York Press, Albany, pp. 65–86.
17. Eisenbach-Stangl, I. (1987) Inebriety and rationality: the modernization of state controls of alcohol-related problems in Austria. *Contemporary Drug Problems* **14**(1), 79–112.
18. Klingemann, H. (1984) Die Rolle der Fachklinik für Alkoholkranke im System interorganisatorischer Zuweisungsprozesse. *Drogen und Alkohol* **3**, 129–147.
19. Eisenbach-Stangl, I. (1999) *Community Action in 'Red Vienna' 1918–1934 – Lessons to be Learned from History*, Paper presented at the First European Symposium on Community Action Programmes to Prevent Alcohol.
20. Parks, K.A. *et al.* (in press) Women's descriptions of drinking in bars: reasons and risks. *Sex Roles*.
21. Mathrani, S. (1995) *Guidelines for City Action on Alcohol*, WHO Regional Office for Europe, Copenhagen.
22. Stockwell, T. *et al.* (1993) High risk drinking settings: the association of serving and promotional practices with harmful drinking. *Addiction* **88**, 1519–1526.
23. Nordhus, G. and Vogt, E. (1981) *Volden og dess ofre* [Violence and its victims]. Cappelens forlag, Oslo.
24. Wells, S. *et al.* (1998) 'The good, the bad and the ugly': responses by security staff to aggressive incidents in public drinking settings. *Journal of Drug Issues* **28**(4), 817–836.
25. Stockwell, T. (1994) Questionnaire for the WHO project on public drinking: Australia.
26. Phipps, A.G. (1999) Applications and effects of geographical research in two quasi-judicial hearings about land-use changes. *Applied Geography* **19**(2), 137–151.
27. Rossow, I. (1996) Alcohol-related violence: the impact of drinking pattern and drinking context. *Addiction* **91**(11), 1651–1661.
28. Dodenhoff, D. (1998) Is welfare really about social control? *Social Service Review* **72**(3), 310–336.
29. Rubington, E. (1977) 'Failure' as a heavy drinker: the case of the chronic-drunkenness offender on Skid Row, in *Society, Culture, and Drinking Patterns* (eds D.J. Pittman and C.R. Snyder), Southern Illinois University Press, Carbondale, Edwardsville, pp. 146–187.
30. Meares, T.L. and Kahan, D.M. (1998) Law and (norms of) order in the inner city. *Law and Society Review* **32**(4), 805–838.
31. Herring, R. (1997) Policy News. Persistent street drinkers: back on the agenda? *Drugs: Education, Prevention and Policy* **4**(2), 187–191.
32. Cox, G.B. *et al.* (1998) Outcome of a controlled trial of the effectiveness of intensive case management for chronic public inebriates. *Journal of Studies on Alcohol* **59**(5), 523–532.
33. Tommasello, A.C. *et al.* (1999) Effectiveness of outreach to homeless substance abusers. *Evaluation and Program Planning* **22**(3), 295–303.
34. Mullahy, J. and Sindelar, J. (1989) Life-cycle effects of alcoholism on education, earnings, and occupation. *Inquiry* **26**, 272–282.
35. Roman, P.M. and Johnson, J.A. (1996) Alcohol's role in work-force entry and retirement. *Alcohol Health and Research World* **20**(3), 162–169.
36. Mullahy, J. and Sindelar, J. (1996) Employment, unemployment and problem drinking. *Journal of Health Economics* **15**, 409–434.

37. Latessa, E.J. et al. (1988) Public support for mandatory drug-alcohol testing in the workplace. *Crime and Delinquency* **34**(4), 379–392.
38. Ames, G.M. and Janes, C. (1990) Drinking, social networks, and the workplace: results of an environmentally focused study, in *Alcohol Problem Intervention in the Workplace: Employee Assistance Programs and Strategic Alternatives* (ed. P.M. Roman), Quorum Books, New York, pp. 95–111.
39. Corsun, D.L. and Young, C.A. (1998) An occupational hazard: alcohol consumption among hospitality managers. *Marriage and Family Review* **28**(1–2), 187–211.
40. Ames, G.M. et al. (1997) The relationship of drinking and hangovers to workplace problems: an empirical study. *Journal of Studies on Alcohol* **58**(1), 37–47.
41. Richman, J.A. et al. (1999) Sexual harassment and generalized workplace abuse among university employees: prevalence and mental health correlates. *American Journal of Public Health* **89**(3), 358–363.
42. Crawford, A. et al. (1987) Unemployment and drinking behaviour: some data from a general population survey of alcohol use. *British Journal of Addiction* **82**, 1007–1016.
43. Hoffmann, J.P. et al. (1996) *Drug Use Among US Workers: Prevalence and Trends by Occupation and Industry Categories*, SAMHSA, Office of Applied Studies, Rockville, MD, (DHHS Publication No. (SMA) 96-3089).
44. Ettner, S.L. (1997) Measuring the human cost of a weak economy: does unemployment lead to alcohol abuse? *Social, Science and Medicine* **4**(2), 251–260.
45. Bongers, I.M.B. et al. (1998) Social climate on alcohol in Rotterdam, the Netherlands: public opinion on drinking behaviour and alcohol control measures. *Alcohol and Alcoholism* **32**(2), 141–150.
46. Single, E. (1997) Public drinking, problems and prevention measures in twelve countries: results of the WHO project on public drinking. *Contemporary Drug Problems* **24**, 425–448.
47. Lenke, L. (1990) *Alcohol and Criminal Violence-Time Series Analyses in a Comparative Perspective*, Almqvist and Wiksell, Stockholm.
48. Süddeutsche Zeitung. (1999) Bayern reagiert auf Urteil. Biergärten sollen bis 23 Uhr offen sein. [Bavaria reacts towards verdict. Beergardens should be open until 11 pm]. *Süddeutsche Zeitung* **02.02**, 8.
49. Gomez-Jacinto, L. and Moral-Toranzo, F. (1999) Urban traffic noise and self-reported health. *Psychological Reports* **84**(3), 1105–1108.
50. Pernanen, K. (1996) *Sammenhengen alkohol-vold* [The Relationship Between Alcohol and Violence], National Institute for Alcohol and Drug Research, Oslo.
51. Marshall, M. and Oleson, A. (1996) MADDer than hell. *Qualitative Health Research* **6**(1), 6–22.
52. McCarthy, J.D. and Wolfson, W. (1996) Resource mobilization by local social movement organizations: agency, strategy and organization in the movement against drinking and driving. *American Sociological Review* **61**(6), 1070–1088.
53. Giesbrecht, N. and Greenfield, T.K. (1999) Public opinions on alcohol policy issues: a comparison of American and Canadian surveys. *Addiction* **94**(4), 521–531.
54. Vowell, P.R. and Howell, F.M. (1998) Modeling delinquent behavior: social disorganization, perceived blocked opportunity, and social control. *Deviant Behavior* **19**(4), 361–395.
55. Room, R. (1999) *Personal communication*.
56. Wechsler, H. et al. (1998) Changes in binge drinking and related problems among American college students between 1993 and 1997 – Results of the Harvard School of Public Health College Alcohol Study. *Journal of American College Health* **47**(2), 57–68.
57. Pavis, S. et al. (1998) Health related behavioural change in context: young people in transition. *Social Science and Medicine* **47**(10), 1407–1418.

58. Back, L. et al. (1999) Beyond the racist/hooligan couplet: race, social theory and football culture. *British Journal of Sociology* **50**(3), 419–442.
59. Verleyen, K. and de Smet, S. (1996) *Hooligans*, Davidsfonds, Leuven.
60. van Limbergen, K. et al. (1989) The societal and psycho-sociological background of football hooliganism. *Current Psychology* **1**, 4–14.

Chapter nine

The social costs of alcohol consumption

E. Gutjahr and G. Gmel

The preceding chapters have shown that alcohol use and misuse can have adverse consequences in such widely differing areas as physical and mental health, traffic safety, violence, and labour productivity. Some entail significant economic costs to society. During the past three decades, considerable efforts have been made to estimate these costs [for an overview, 1–3]. Recent investigations suggest that they represent annually a substantial part of the Gross Domestic Product of industrialized countries.

The present chapter reviews some of the literature and outlines the magnitude of social costs of alcohol consumption in Europe. It is organized around the following issues:

- What constitutes social costs and how they are estimated
- Recent European and non-European estimates
- Policy implications

WHAT CONSTITUTES SOCIAL COSTS AND HOW THEY ARE ESTIMATED

Alcohol consumption has adverse consequences for health and social life. The chronic effects on health such as various neoplasms or liver cirrhosis are, in general, well documented in the scientific literature [for an overview, 4, 5–9]. Less is known, however, about the acute health effects, such as various injuries resulting from traffic accidents, falls etc., or about the social consequences.

Harald Klingemann and Gerhard Gmel (eds.), Mapping the Social Consequences of Alcohol Consumption, 133–143.
© *2001 Kluwer Academic Publishers. Printed in Great Britain.*

Nevertheless, there is growing evidence on the relationship between alcohol and crime (see chapter Chapter 8), violent behaviour (Chapter 6), suicide (Chapter 7) and workplace problems (Chapter 5). On the assumption that the adverse consequences of drinking can be evaluated in monetary terms, health scientists and economists have attempted to estimate the costs of alcohol consumption to society.

Basic questions of cost analysis are: what constitutes costs and what are social costs? To begin with the latter question, social costs are largely defined as costs to society, i.e. all costs arising from alcohol consumption that are not borne exclusively, knowingly and freely by the drinker, such as spending on the drinks [10, 11]. Thus, social costs are the negative economic impact of alcohol consumption on the material welfare of society.

In defining costs, a key distinction is made between direct and indirect costs. According to Harwood *et al.* [2], direct costs refer to the value of goods and services actually delivered to address the harmful effects of alcohol consumption. In contrast, indirect costs represent the value of personal productive services that are not performed because of the adverse consequences of drinking. The major categories of cost analysis are shown in Table 1.

Consequences to the health system include all monetary costs of dealing with alcohol misuse and dependence as well as alcohol-related diseases or injuries, irrespective of the specific provider of treatment (hospital, clinic, physician, ambulance). Welfare service costs include the costs of administering social-assistance and counselling programmes as well as public and private insurance benefits. They comprise, in addition, the costs of initial and continuing education of professionals, such as alcohol-abuse counsellors, mental health professionals and clergy, in the care and management of individuals with alcohol-related diseases or problems. The costs of judicial system services includes essentially those of law enforcement, judicial proceedings and correction (prison). Alcohol consumption can lead to material damage, especially through traffic accidents, workplace accidents, offences such as assault, and arson.

Furthermore, alcohol use and misuse has a major impact on the workplace (Chapter 5). It affects not only the supply of labour but also labour productivity. Primarily, alcohol-related costs arise from premature death, excess unemployment and absenteeism, as well as from work accidents and reduced efficiency on the job due to morbidity (illnesses, hangovers, reduced motor-skills, etc.) [12, 13–23]. According to the human capital approach, it is assumed that a healthy human being represents for society a value equal to the productivity which that human being can achieve during his or her active life. Consequently, indirect costs are the sum of the individual salaries that are lost because of excess illness, impaired functioning and premature mortality [2, 10, 24].

Table 1 Overview of the cost items generally included in social-cost studies of alcohol consumption

---

Direct costs

Direct core costs – costs to health, judicial and social welfare systems
Medical care
- hospital treatment of alcohol-related diseases and injuries
- outpatient treatment provided by services and office-based physicians
- pharmaceuticals

Welfare system services
- social assistance and counselling
- administration of insurance benefits
- professional education, prevention and research

Judicial system services
- police, fire brigades and rescue operations
- court work
- prison services

Direct non-core costs – related costs due to material damage
Material damage
- due to accidents
- due to offences (burglary, assault, etc.)
- due to fire

Indirect costs

Costs due to productivity losses
Premature mortality (person years of life lost)
Excess unemployment and excess morbidity

RECENT EUROPEAN AND NON-EUROPEAN COST ESTIMATES

Most of the literature on social costs of alcohol consumption is from the English-speaking, non-European countries, especially from the United States of America, Canada, New Zealand and Australia [see the reports 2, 19, 25–30]. Rooted in a strong tradition, studies in those countries employ elaborate methods and data. Also, European studies are usually limited in scope to only a few selected cost items for which empirical data are easily available. There are, nevertheless, some valuable studies, which are presented globally in this chapter and compared with the non-European literature. First, however, a Finnish investigation [31] is presented and discussed in some detail (Table 2). It is one of the most recent European studies to take up the state of the art in methods of estimating social costs of alcohol consumption.

Table 2 Estimates of the social costs of alcohol misuse in Finland in 1990

Cost items/value	US$ (millions)[a]	% of total costs
Direct core costs	636–853	15.0–19.0
Medical care	287–401	7.00–8.6
Hospital treatment	216–266	4.67–6.45
Outpatient treatment	Not estimated	Not estimated
Pharmaceuticals	Not estimated	Not estimated
Disability pensions	71–135	2.1–2.4
Welfare system services	108–139	2.4–3.2
Social-assistance and counselling programmes	71–102	1.8–2.1
Administration of insurance benefits	Not estimated	Not estimated
Professional education, prevention and research	37–37	0.67–1.1
Judicial system services	241–313	5.5–7.23
Police, fire brigades and rescue operations	114–154	2.7–3.4
Courts	109–136	2.4–3.3
Prisons	18–23	0.4–0.5
Other direct costs	110–123	2.1–3.3
Material damage	110–123	2.1–3.3
due to traffic accidents	37–46	0.8–1.1
due to offences (e.g. assault)	73–77	1.3–2.2
due to fire	Not estimated	Not estimated
Indirect costs	2605–4762	77.7–83.0
Premature mortality	2459–4598	73.4–80.1
Excess morbidity	146–164	2.9–4.4
Total costs	3351–5738	100.0

Source: Salomaa [31]
[a] lower and upper estimates as indicated in the original report

Depending upon the basic assumptions, viz. whether they are more or less conservative (i.e. cautious in the attribution of social harm, and its extent, to alcohol) the estimated total costs of alcohol consumption amount to between 2% and 4% of the gross domestic product (GDP) of Finland. Medical care for alcohol-related diseases and injuries costs no more than one fifth of the total costs. Nevertheless, the numbers of hospital episodes and hospital bed days are high. In 1990, about 15 000 patients received hospital treatment for alcohol-related illnesses. Between 170 000 and 270 000 hospital bed days were attributable to alcohol-related diseases such as alcoholism, psychosis, and diseases of the liver, and almost as many to alcohol-related accidents and acts of violence.

In Finland, the number of treatment periods and hospital bed days in 1990 was:

- 175 000–275 000 for alcohol-related illnesses
- 159 000–242 000 for alcohol-related accidents and acts of violence

Total: 334 000–517 000 hospital bed-days (3.2–4.9% of all bed-days

Source: Salomaa [31]

The costs of alcohol use and misuse to the Finnish judicial system, viz. police interventions, and court and rescue services, clearly exceeded those of medical care. The principal cost items were maintenance of order, traffic control, investigations and searches, as well as police duty. Alcohol-related cases accounted for more than 20% of the tasks undertaken by the police. The very high costs of law enforcement and judicial proceedings may, however, be particular to Finland. In some of the Nordic countries, legislation on drinking in public places requires the police to arrest intoxicated persons who are no longer able to look after themselves or who constitute a danger to others (Chapter 8). In contrast to the high costs of police and judicial-system services, expenditure on education, prevention and research does not exceed 1% of the total alcohol-related costs.

The most serious economic consequences of alcohol consumption are to the workplace – to labour supply and productivity. In Finland in 1990, about 2400 alcohol-related deaths were reported, of which about 25% were ascribed to alcohol-related illnesses, more than 25% to intentional violence (mostly suicide, but also homicides), and more than 40% to accidents. These deaths resulted in a reduction of the labour force, at least in the case of the individuals in the active-life period who were not already incapacitated by alcohol.

In Finland, in 1990, alcohol-related deaths numbered:

- 670–720 from alcohol-related illnesses
- 600–630 from intentional violence (2/3 suicides)
- 1030–1150 from accidents

Source: Salomaa [31]

The number of person years of life years lost, not presented in the Finnish study, may be roughly estimated. Given that deaths from alcohol-related diseases occur mostly at older ages (60 years and over) as serious diseases develop only over a long period of drinking, that alcohol-related intentional violence tends to occur in the middle-aged (30–50 years), and that most alcohol-related accidents occur at younger ages (20–30), it can be estimated that the 2400 alcohol-related deaths result in about 20 000 to 25 000 person years of life lost. The value of each person year of life lost equals the value of the mean annual pay of an employed person or, for those persons not in the labour force, the value imputed for one year of private domestic services.

The results of the Finnish study correspond roughly with those from a wider, international background. Table 3 gives an overview of the results of some selected studies of both European and non-European origin.

The table shows that, despite the common theoretical framework of the studies, the total estimated costs vary greatly. The range, expressed as share of GDP, extends from 0.25% to 5.73%. All but one of the studies presented in Table 3 indicate that indirect costs outweigh direct costs. What is particularly costly to society is, thus, not so much medical care for alcohol-related illness or material damages from traffic accidents, but, rather, the consequences to national productivity in terms of person years of life lost, excess unemployment and reduced work-performance [10, 21].

Table 3 reveals also that, except for the Finnish investigation, the European cost studies suggest strikingly lower total cost figures, hardly exceeding 0.5% of GDP [32–34], compared with the non-European estimates of between 1.1% and 5.7% of GDP. This is due basically to the use of different methods. As a matter of fact, most European investigators estimate only some selected cost items, not the entire array set out in Table 1. Reasons invoked for this restriction are lack of, or difficulty in obtaining, relevant data and insufficient funds for realizing a broader scope of investigation. Since European studies tend to underestimate considerably the social costs of alcohol consumption, a look at results from a wider international background is required. Under the assumption that (a) the results of the non-European investigations constitute a reliable basis from the theoretical and methodological as well as the empirical points of view, and that, (b) the social costs of alcohol consumption in Europe do not differ fundamentally from those in the United States, Canada, New Zealand and Australia, it may be concluded that estimates for Europe should correspond roughly with the non-European and Finnish examples. Thus, from the available evidence, average cost figures can be inferred both globally in terms of total costs and more precisely in terms of direct and indirect costs:

Table 3 Overview of cost estimates from various countries

Year of data	1992[b]	1985[c]	1992[d]	Cost estimates (millions of US$)[a] 1991[e]	1990[f]	1994[g]	1990[h]	1983[i]
Direct costs	41 024	18 900	3385	341–589	746–976	3763–4325	958	331
Indirect costs	106 997	51 400	4137	704–3389	2605–4762	3615–4155	2730	2116
Total costs	148 021	70 300	7522	1045–3978	3351–5738	7378–8480	3688	2447
Total costs relative to GDP (%)	2.3	1.7	1.1	1.5–5.7	2–4	0.67–0.77	0.25	0.5
Share of direct costs in total costs	27.7	26.9	45.0	14.8–32.6	17.0–22.3	51.0–51.0	26.0	13.5
Share of indirect costs in total costs	72.3	73.1	55.0	67.4–85.2	77.7–83.0	49.0–49.0	74.0	86.5

[a]At constant prices and exchange rates of 1990
[b]Harwood et al., USA [2]; [c]Rice et al., USA [24]; [d]Single et al., Canada [26]; [e]Devlin et al., New Zealand [27]; [f]Salomaa, Finland [31]; [g]Collicelli, Italy [33]; [h]Brecht, Germany [32]; [i]McDonnell and Maynard, UK [34]

- The social costs of alcohol consumption amount to between 1% and 3% of GDP;
- For the European Union[1] in 1998, the social costs of alcohol consumption can be estimated at between US$ 64 939 and 194 817 million;[2]
- About 20% of the total costs (US$ 15 990–47 971 million) are direct costs, representing the amount actually spent for medical, social and judicial services;
- About 10% of the total costs (US$ 7995–23 986 million) are spent for material damage;
- About 70% of the total costs (US$ 55 966–167 899 million) represent lost earnings of individuals unable to perform their productive tasks in the way they would had they not been consuming alcohol.

Even though these figures are hypothetical, they nevertheless have a solid empirical foundation, namely results of major cost studies conducted recently and applying an elaborate costing methodology. Their chief advantage is that they provide rough indicators which can be applied to any country or any year. Their corresponding disadvantage is that they do not take account of cross-cultural differences in drinking patterns or of demographic and epidemiological variations. In fact, not only drinking patterns but also social and cultural norms affect the relationship between alcohol consumption and adverse outcomes (Chapter 8). It may be assumed, therefore, that costs vary equally across cultures. As the Finnish study has shown, national features such as the rigid legal responses to alcohol-related social behaviour in Finland, can add greatly to the social costs.

The literature so far, however, does not provide culture-specific estimations. This remains a major challenge to research.

POLICY IMPLICATIONS

The past decade has seen growing interest in social-cost analysis on the part not only of health-care providers and addiction specialists, but also of politicians determined to reduce the adverse consequences of alcohol consumption.

---

[1] Austria, Belgium, Denmark, Finland, France, Germany, Greece, Ireland, Italy, Luxembourg, Netherlands, Portugal, Spain, Sweden, United Kingdom.
[2] At constant prices and exchange rates of 1990.

Estimates of social costs provide an indicator of the overall economic burden of alcohol use and misuse to a given society. Since cost analysis not only results in an overall figure but also provides detailed estimates of financial consequences for the health, welfare and judicial systems, and even for the workplace, it enables policy-makers to single out the key areas where alcohol harms the social and material welfare of society and to develop policy measures specifically for those areas.

Social cost studies, however, are not studies of the impact of alcohol consumption on national budgets. They refer to costs to society as a whole. Also, unlike studies of budgetary impact, they do not usually take account of tax revenues or other benefits such as employment in the production and distribution of alcohol. Neither does cost analysis provide information on cost-effectiveness of any policy measures adopted. Politicians need this kind of information to guide their decisions between different options and set priorities in public-health policy on alcohol. Cost analysis has still to develop adequate ways of evaluating cost-effectiveness.

For policy-makers, comparison of social costs of alcohol consumption with government expenditures on health, education and social welfare may be of interest. For this purpose, three examples of countries from Northern, Southern and Central Europe have been chosen (see Table 4). For Eastern Europe, no consolidated national accounts are yet available. The figures representing the estimated social costs of alcohol consumption in Table 4 are inferential and based on the assumption that those costs amount to between 1% and 3% of the GDP of each country.

Table 4 Comparison of some selected components of national budgets, 1990

	Norway[a]	France[b]	Germany[c] (Federal Republic)
Estimated social costs of alcohol consumption (lower and upper estimates = 1–3% of GDP)	6629–19888	67665–202995	27820–83460
Government final consumption expenditures by function in current prices			
Health	31229	215260	136500
Education	35722	324163	84070
Social security and welfare	13860	92206	53160
Total Government final consumption expenditure	139115	1238998	444070

Source: United Nations [35] and OECD [36–38]
[a]Norwegian kroner (million); [b]French francs (million); [c]Deutsche marks (million)

Table 4 shows that, for the selected European countries, the estimated social costs of alcohol consumption are comparable to, or even exceed, government expenditures on social security and welfare, and approximate one fourth of that on health. Clearly, the adverse consequences of alcohol use and misuse are significant and call for policy measures to reduce them. The chapters that follow deal with the key issues of how policy action may reduce harm and what local community action has achieved.

REFERENCES

1. ICAP. (1999) *Estimating Costs Associated with Alcohol Abuse: Towards a Patterns Approach*, International Center of Alcohol Policies, Washington, DC, (ICAP Report).
2. Harwood, H., Fountain, D. and Livermore, G. (1998) *The Economic Costs of Alcohol and Drug Abuse in the United States, 1992*, US Department of Health and Human Services, National Institute on Drug Abuse, Rockville, MD, (NIH Publication Number 98-4327).
3. Sindelar, J. (1998) Social costs of alcohol. *Journal of Drug Issues* **28**(3), 763–780.
4. Single, E., Robson, L., Rehm, J. and Xie, X. (1999) Morbidity and mortality attributable to alcohol, tobacco, and illicit drug use in Canada. *American Journal of Public Health* **89**(3), 385–390.
5. Rehm, J., Ashley, M.J. and Dubois, G. (1996) Alcohol and health: individual and population perspectives. *Addiction* **92**, S109–S115.
6. Edwards, G., Anderson, P., Babor, T.F. et al. (1994) *Alcohol Policy and the Public Good*, Oxford University Press, Oxford.
7. United States Department of Health and Human Services (1997) *Ninth Special Report to the US Congress on Alcohol and Health from the Secretary of Health and Human Services*, US Department of Health and Human Services, Public Health Service, National Institutes of Health, National Institute on Alcohol Abuse and Alcoholism, Washington (NIH Publication No. 97-4017).
8. English, D.R., Holman, C.D.J., Milne, E., Winter, M.G., Hulse, G.K. and Codde, J.P. (1995) *The Quantification of Drug Caused Morbidity and Mortality in Australia*, Commonwealth Department of Human Services and Health, Canberra.
9. Stinson, F.S. and DeBakey, S.M. (1992) Alcohol-related mortality in the United States, 1979–1988. *British Journal of Addiction* **87**, 777–783.
10. Godfrey, C. (1997) Lost productivity and costs to society. *Addiction* **92**(Suppl 1), S49–S54.
11. Single, E., Collins, D., Easton, B., Harwood, H., Lapsley, H. and Maynard, A. (1996) *International Guidelines for Estimating the Social Costs of Substance Abuse*, Canadian Centre on Substance Abuse, Toronto.
12. Ames, G.M., Grube, J.W. and Moore, R.S. (1997) The relationship of drinking and hangovers to workplace problems: an empirical study. *Journal of Studies on Alcohol* **58**(1), 37–47.
13. Blum, T.C., Roman, P.M. and Martin, J.K. (1993) Alcohol consumption and work performance. *Journal of Studies on Alcohol* **54**, 61–70.
14. Hollo, C.D., Leigh, J. and Nurminen, M. (1993) Role of alcohol in work-related fatal accidents in Australia 1982–1984. *Occupational Medicine* **43**, 13–17.
15. International Labour Office (ILO). (1998) *Substance Abuse and the Workplace: Current State of Research and Future Needs*, International Labour Office, Geneva.

16. Jones, S., Casswell, S. and Zhang, J.F. (1995) The economic costs of alcohol related absenteeism and reduced productivity among the working population of New Zealand. *Addiction* **90**, 1455–1461.
17. Mangione, T.W., Howland, J., Amick, B. et al. (1999) Employee drinking practices and work performance. *Journal of Studies on Alcohol* **60**, 261–270.
18. Single, E. (1998) *Substance Abuse and the Workplace in Canada*, Canadian Centre on Substance Abuse, Ottawa, (Report prepared for Health Canada on behalf of the Canadian Centre on Substance Abuse).
19. Heien, D. and Pittman, D.J. (1989) The economic costs of alcohol abuse: an assessment of current methods and estimates. *Journal of Studies on Alcohol* **50**(6), 567–579.
20. Mullahy, J. and Sindelar, J. (1992) Effects of alcohol on labor market success. *Alcohol Health and Research World* **16**(2), 134–139.
21. Mullahy, J. and Sindelar, J. (1996) Employment, unemployment and problem drinking. *Journal of Health Economics* **15**, 409–434.
22. Mullahy, J. and Sindelar, J. (1998) Drinking, problem drinking and productivity. *Recent Developments in Alcoholism* **14**, 347–359.
23. French, M.T. and Zarkin, G.A. (1995) Is moderate alcohol use related to wages? Evidence from four worksites. *Journal of Health Economics* **14**, 319–344.
24. Rice, D.P., Kelman, S., Miller, L.S. and Dunmeyer, S. (1990) *The Economic Costs of Alcohol and Drug Abuse and Mental Illness: 1985*, Report submitted to the Alcohol, Drug Abuse, and Mental Health Administration, US Department of Health and Human Services. Institute for Health and Aging, University of California, San Francisco, CA (DHHS Publication No. (ADM) 90-1694).
25. Single, E., Robson, L.S., Xie, X. and Rehm, J.T. (1998) The economic costs of alcohol, tobacco and illicit drugs in Canada, 1992. *Addiction* **93**(7), 991–1006.
26. Single, E., Robson, L., Xie, X. and Rehm, J. (1996) *The Costs of Substance Abuse in Canada*, Canadian Centre on Substance Abuse, Ottawa, Ontario.
27. Devlin, N.J., Scuffham, P.A. and Bunt, L.J. (1997) The social costs of alcohol abuse in New Zealand. *Addiction* **92**(11), 1491–1505.
28. Collins, D. and Lapsley, H. (1996) *The Social Costs of Drug Abuse in Australia in 1988 and 1992*, Commonwealth Department of Human Services and Health, Canberra.
29. Collins, D. and Lapsley, H. (1991) *Estimating the Economic Costs of Drug Abuse in Australia*, Commonwealth of Australia, (No. 15), Canberra.
30. Robson, L. and Single, E. (1995) *Literature Review of Studies on the Economic Costs of Substance Abuse*, Canadian Centre on Substance Abuse, Ottawa.
31. Salomaa, J. (1995) The costs of the detrimental effects of alcohol abuse have grown faster than alcohol consumption in Finland. *Addiction* **90**, 525–537.
32. Brecht, J.G., Poldrugo, F. and Schädlich, P.K. (1996) Alcoholism – The cost of illness in the Federal Republic of Germany. *PharmacoEconomics* **10**(5), 484–493.
33. Collicelli, C. (1996) Income from alcohol and the costs of alcoholism: an Italian experience. *Alcologia* **8**(2), 135–143.
34. McDonnell, R. and Maynard, A. (1985) The costs of alcohol misuse. *British Journal of Addiction* **80**, 27–35.
35. United Nations. (1997) *National Accounts Statistics: Main Aggregates and Detailed Tables, 1994–Part I*, United Nations, Department for Economic and Social Information and Policy Analysis, Statistics Division, New York.
36. OECD. (1992) *OECD Economic Surveys – France*, Organisation for Economic Co-Operation and Development, Paris Cedex.
37. OECD. (1992) *OECD Economic Surveys – Norway*, Organisation for Economic Co-Operation and Development, Paris Cedex.
38. OECD. (1992) *OECD Economic Surveys – Germany*, Organisation for Economic Co-Operation and Development, Paris Cedex.

Chapter ten

Harm minimization

M. Plant

INTRODUCTION: WHAT IS 'HARM MINIMIZATION'?

The control of alcohol-related problems is an intensely political and contentious subject, involving a host of interests that often promote entirely different agendas. Some of the most hotly debated issues include such topics as the use of taxation and restrictions on the availability of alcoholic beverages [1]. In general terms, any policy intended to reduce the level of alcohol-related problems, such as public disorder, accidents, injuries, illness and premature death, could loosely be termed 'harm minimization'. Indeed, as recently noted by Single [2], one individual has claimed that the 'harm minimization' of illicit drug problems included the incarceration of drug users. Many would view this as a drastic and unacceptable step. In fact, there has for some time been a clear division between what is currently termed 'harm minimization' or 'harm reduction' and a rather different, but equally legitimate, approach, which has been called the 'public health perspective' in relation to alcohol and its associated problems. It is a contention of this chapter that these two approaches are not in essence so very different, even though they have sometimes been presented as being 'rival' perspectives. Moreover, it is stressed that harm minimization and the public health perspective are neither mutually exclusive nor incompatible. Throughout the past two centuries, national and regional approaches to curbing alcohol-related problems have ranged from attempts to stamp out drinking completely (NB Prohibition) to measures designed to deal with specific manifestations of the harmful consumption of alcohol [3]. During the past 25 years there have been several publications that have attempted to set out a general theoretical and practical perspective on the vexed issue of 'what to do about alcohol'. This topic continues to have considerable importance and is

Harald Klingemann and Gerhard Gmel (eds.), Mapping the Social Consequences of Alcohol Consumption, 145–160.
© *2001 Kluwer Academic Publishers. Printed in Great Britain.*

inevitably complex because alcohol, a hugely popular psychoactive substance, may be used harmfully or, in moderation, in a beneficial manner [4]. Bruun et al. [5] produced an important and influential report, *Alcohol Control Policies in Public Health Perspective*. This gave great emphasis to the assertion that, as noted by Ledermann [6], rates of alcohol-related problems, such as liver cirrhosis mortality, are associated with per capita alcohol consumption. Accordingly, the key to curbing rates of alcohol-related problems is to control alcohol consumption in general. This view was reaffirmed by Kreitman [7], who stressed a 'preventive paradox', namely the fact that there are far more light and intermediate drinkers than heavy drinkers. Accordingly, it is important to reduce the alcohol consumption of the majority who do not drink heavily to achieve any major impact on the general population level of alcohol consumption and in so doing to reduce problems. A broadly similar view has since been expounded by several other authors, such as Edwards et al. [8] and by the World Health Organization [9]. This approach has been light-heartedly called 'draining the ocean to prevent shark attacks' [10]. It may be useful at this stage to draw attention to a parallel debate in connection with policies to deal with illicit drugs, especially since the advent of HIV/AIDS and hepatitis C amongst injecting drug users. The illogic, racism, homophobia and other injustices of past drug and HIV/AIDS policies have been brilliantly reviewed by Schilts and Gray [11, 12]. Broadly, approaches to illicit drug use have polarized into a 'zero tolerance' or drug-use eradication approach and an alternative perspective, namely harm minimization or harm reduction. It is clear that attempts to eradicate drug use have not been successful; even 'primary prevention'/health promotion, designed to discourage young people from trying drugs, has a very poor record of achievement [13].

Harm minimization or harm reduction approaches to illicit drugs attempt to curb, not necessarily drug use per se, but harmful drug use and the damaging consequences of dangerous forms of drug use. Harm minimization has encompassed such strategies as the distribution of sterile injecting equipment and of condoms and the operation of Methadone maintenance programmes [14–17].

As noted, a number of commentators have advocated a similar harm-reduction or harm-minimization approach to alcohol control policies [10, 18, 19]. They have argued, not for the reduction of per capita alcohol consumption as a prime policy aim, but for the adoption of measures to reduce levels of specific types of alcohol-related harm. The value of this more closely targeted approach has been strengthened by a growing body of evidence that suggests that the social consequences of drinking are associated with patterns of alcohol consumption among sub-groups of drinkers [20]. Moreover, rates of alcohol-related problems, including social consequences, are not uniform. Sometimes such rates may move in quite different ways and even go in opposite directions [4]. In relation to alcohol, 'harm minimization' has been briefly summed up thus:

'avoid problems when you drink'. [19, *op cit.* p. 7]

In fact, the types of policy and approach that advocates of either a 'public health' or a 'harm minimization' approach have been promoting are largely much the same.

In most parts of the world, governments appear not to have been eager to adjust per capita alcohol consumption levels as a control policy, presumably for political and economic reasons. Accordingly, more specific measures have been used. As Greenfield and Kaskutas [21] and Greenfield [22] have noted with reference to evidence from the United States, public support for controls is greatest for the options that are least likely to influence individuals, such as the use of warning labels and health education. One example of a harm-reduction approach is provided by a recent report from the Northern Ireland Department of Health and Social Services [23]. It sets out a policy agenda based upon the following perspective:

'targeting specific risk behaviours (e.g. 'binge drinking') through a co-ordinated approach including health promotion, treatment and enforcement rather than concentrating on consumption levels alone'. (p.ii)

It goes on to suggest a number of specific policies to curb alcohol problems among specific groups of drinkers, such as young people, older people and women.

Is there any practical and pragmatic way of judging the value of 'harm minimization' strategies? Reiterating earlier work by Plant, Single and Stockwell [19, *op cit.* p. 263], it is suggested that the specific policy options that are available or have been used to reduce levels of alcohol-related harm should be assessed in relation to the following four considerations:

- Have they worked?
- Are they transferable to other contexts?
- Are they politically and socially acceptable?
- Can they be sustained?

This chapter attempts to provide a brief and highly selective introduction to a number of different ways in which attempts have been made to curb the adverse consequences of alcohol consumption.

EDUCATION

One of the most popular and least intrusive alcohol policy options is health education or health promotion. Considerable effort has been invested in education, especially in relation to teenagers and school-age children. Much of this activity has been well-intentioned but it has had no clear objectives, and relatively few such initiatives have ever been evaluated. Nevertheless, the evaluative literature is now considerable [13, 24]. The most striking conclusion from the available evidence is that neither alcohol education nor health promotion has succeeded in modifying youthful drinking patterns. This conclusion holds true even with reference to some of the most ambitious and expensive ventures in this field. In particular, the United States police-based 'DARE' (Drug Abuse Resistance), and the Australian 'Life Education' programmes have failed to discourage young people from using alcohol, tobacco or illicit drugs [25–27]. From the Australian initiative, evidence has emerged suggesting that it may have raised rather than reduced levels of psychoactive drug use [28]. Taken overall, evidence suggests that alcohol education may raise levels of knowledge and may also change attitudes, though often for only a short period. Alcohol education may, of course, serve several objectives apart from changing drinking behaviour (which has been difficult to achieve by education alone). It may, for example, be used to inform the public or specific groups, such as politicians, health care professionals, young people, drivers or pregnant women, about policy issues, or provide factual information, or be a valuable complement to other harm-minimization strategies, such as community-based or national campaigns. As noted later in this chapter, the use of warning labels, one form of education, has achieved some tangible results [24, 29].

Education has been able to raise awareness, increase knowledge and change attitudes, and has done so in different settings. Alcohol education has a high degree of political support but needs to be sustained to produce lasting effects.

COMMUNITY ACTION

As recently noted by Allamani *et al.* [30], there have been a large number of instances of 'community action' designed to deal with problems that have caused special concern. Madden and Thornton [31], in relation to a study of deprived Scottish communities, have reported that problems related to alcohol may emerge as important local issues. These may include public intoxication and disorder or noise around late-night drinking venues. The responses to such problems have been varied, ranging from the installation of video surveillance cameras in 'trouble spots', such as outside bars, night clubs and town centres in which people may gather in the evening and during the night time, to local by-laws permitting bans on public drinking in specified areas. The introduction of video surveillance in the town of Stornoway, on the Scottish island of Lewis, has 'quietened things down', though no formal data appear to be available on recorded crime levels or other variables [32]. Also, new by-laws banning public drinking in certain specified areas in Scottish towns and cities have led to a fall in alcohol-related problems in the localities concerned [32, 33]. One factor that needs to be considered in relation to the impact of any specific local policy is 'displacement': does the introduction of a policy intended to deal with a problem simply move the problem to another, less controlled, area? Many of these types of measures have been introduced in the United Kingdom and other countries but, regrettably, there have been only a few published assessments of their impact. There have, fortunately, been several exceptions to this lack of documentation.

Jeffs and Saunders [34] have described an experiment introduced by the police in the English coastal town of Torquay, a popular tourist resort. Reacting to concern about intoxication and disorder in and around harbour-area bars, the police introduced a policy of rigorously enforcing the licensing laws. Uniformed police officers maintained a conspicuous presence in the target area, having visited bars and informed their owners and managers that they would not tolerate infringements of the law (such as serving people who were intoxicated or under age, or remaining open outside permitted hours). During a trial period of one year, alcohol-related crime fell by over 20%. Some other forms of crime also declined. There was no evidence to suggest that this policy had displaced problems to other areas. The drop in crime in Torquay contrasted with rising crime in a comparison town during the same period. This experiment showed how, simply by enforcing current laws, a local initiative could achieve a major improvement, in the case of Torquay a highly successful outcome. Strangely, it seems that this experiment was not sustained, nor did the police in other parts of Britain adopt it. Only one force, in Sussex, appears to have attempted to adopt the 'Torquay approach'. Two Scottish police forces report success in reducing rates of alcohol-related crime with a similar, vigorous enforcement, approach [35, 36]. A major factor in this apparent lack of interest has been that alcohol is often not a high priority in relation to other issues, such as violent crime, motor-vehicle theft, burglary or illicit drugs. This may appear paradoxical, since heavy drinking is clearly associated with many forms of criminal activity [37].

Another example of the use of concerted community action has been reported in relation to an Australian 'Gold Coast' town known as 'Surfers Paradise', which had the same problems as those that had motivated the Torquay experiment, namely intoxication, violence and disorder. Particular concern focused on an area that included 28 night-clubs surrounding a place called Cavill Mall. In response to what has been described as 'panic' about safety and security in this area, the Surfers Paradise Safety Action Plan was initiated as a result of strong pressures from worried local business people. Saltz [38, p. 81] has described this in the following words:

'The programme comprised three major strategies: the development of community-based task forces, conducting risk assessment similar to those done in Freemantle, with subsequent implementation of a community 'code of practice', and increased enforcement of licence laws, particularly those tied to the prevention of assaults. Training was offered, primarily to security staff, in ways to deal with patron intoxication, and the code of practice emphasised refusal of service to intoxicated patrons, along with responsible advertising and, most importantly perhaps, the elimination of free drinks and extreme price promotions'.

Homel and Clark [39] and Homel *et al.* [40], cited by Saltz [38], concluded that there had been a significant decrease in assaults in a sample of alcoholic beverage outlets after this project commenced. Observational research also indicated a reduction in both intoxication and binge drinking among men. The local police reported a fall in rates of violence and other crimes in the target area, while they continued to rise in other parts of the town. These results have been considered by Graham and Homel [41]:

'A key element in the project was that it provided a structure for focusing the community militancy about safety and security by channelling energy into a Steering Committee, three major task groups, and a Monitoring Committee responsible for overseeing adherence to a code of practice developed by night club managers'. (p. 184)

A third, and very important, example of community action on alcohol has been provided by the Lahti Project [42]. This initiative, which, unusually, was inspired by alcohol researchers, involved a battery of interventions that were carried out in a Finnish city between 1993 and 1994. These were designed to increase the knowledge of primary care professionals about alcohol-related issues, the staging of educational events, youth work, counselling sessions for families, sales surveillance, and server training for bar staff. Moreover, this ambitious exercise set out to create new networks among welfare professionals and others, and to influence the 'alcohol policy thinking' of key people and of the researchers.

This study did not transform local drinking habits, but this is not surprising. It did, however, raise the profile of alcohol issues in Lahti. Newspaper reports on the prevention of alcohol problems increased. Most of the local population knew of events organized by the project team, and the public became more aware of alcohol as a social problem and more knowledgeable about alcohol. Popular support for the use of public funds for the prevention of alcohol problems also increased, and social services providing counselling and support for problem drinkers were extended and improved. These were all positive and worthwhile results.

Holmila has provided the following thoughtful and invaluable comment on the outcome of the Lahti exercise:

'The main lesson from the project can, perhaps, be formulated in the following way: the type of community prevention that really works and creates sustainable changes is neither value-neutral nor given from above; rather, it is ritualistic and, emotional and requires subjective involvement of the people in the community. This is not to say that prevention needs to be irrational. But its rationality should not be of the limited kind'. [42, p. 216]

Moskalewicz and Swiatkiewicz [43] have described a community action project at Malczyce, Poland. This led to the production of booklets and videos to aid communities in their prevention efforts. The authors concluded that factors contributing to the sustainability of a community project could be identified and analysed through the use of simple community surveys and focus groups. The projects at Lahti and Malczyce are discussed in more detail in Chapter 11. These initiatives were clearly able to achieve some, albeit limited, harm-minimization objectives. They also lend support to the need to sustain such ventures if any tangible gains are to be maintained.

Several lessons emerge from the examples of Torquay, Surfers Paradise, Lahti and Malczyce. The first is that effective community action usually begins when a key person, or a group of influential people, creates a well-motivated coalition of individuals. These may have very different backgrounds but must have a shared concern. Secondly, even if local action to reduce alcohol problems is 'effective' in some clear and tangible way, impact needs to be publicized, not just once but repeatedly; otherwise interest and commitment may wane and the effective policy may be abandoned. The issue of 'sustainability' is discussed later in this chapter. Thirdly, even short-term community action can effectively highlight local concerns about the social consequences of drinking.

Community action has been shown to reduce public nuisance, crime and disorder, to raise awareness of alcohol issues and to improve the provision of alcohol services. Some strategies may be transferable to other settings, but such initiatives require local public and political support. Sadly, few such community initiatives appear to have been sustained.

SAFER DRINKING-PLACES

The possibility that drinking places, such as bars, might be made safer has attracted much interest. The classic work of Graham [44] in Vancouver bars suggested that the lay-out, design and organization of such locales were associated with levels of both intoxication and aggression among patrons. This connection gives rise to a number of possible options designed to reduce such undesirable aspects of the public drinking scene. This has been discussed earlier by Graham et al. [45], Graham and Homel [41] and Graham and Plant [46]. An intriguing body of evidence has been produced on the subject of drinking in bars [47]. Some of it suggests that situational factors may influence bar-room-drinking [48]. Factors shown to be associated with patrons' drinking patterns include the speed of country music played in a bar (slower tempo was related to faster drinking) [49], and being touched by waitresses (this was associated with higher consumption) [50].

One example of a non-intrusive way to make bars safer is the use of toughened drinking glasses. 'Normal' drinking glasses break into dagger-like shards and inflict injury either accidentally or by use in deliberate assaults. Shepherd, a surgeon, and colleagues [51, 52] drew attention to the possibility of using tempered or toughened glasses. Pilot research by Plant *et al.* [53] and Plant and Mills [54] has supported this view. It has suggested that toughened glasses, though a little more expensive than the non-toughened variety, are much stronger and less liable to break into dangerous fragments, and cause fewer injuries when used in bars. They may be used also for drinking in the home, in restaurants and cafes, at work or in other places as well as in bars.

Graham and Homel [41] have suggested a number of other ways to make bars safer. They include the types of server training scheme and responsible beverage service that have already been cited above in relation to Surfers Paradise and Lahti.

Clearly, drinking places can be made safer by reducing both intoxication and aggression. Ways of doing this vary according to local and national sentiment. Once more, it is emphasizsed that successful measures need to be sustained to retain lasting value.

LABELLING TO WARN AND INFORM

Labels have been used in a number of ways to form or warn drinkers about alcohol-related issues. A well-known example of this has been the introduction of warnings on alcohol containers and at sales outlets in the USA. These have been reviewed in detail by Greenfield [22]. Similar warning labels have been introduced in India and Mexico. The United States warnings, as noted by Greenfield [22, *op cit.* p. 106], were introduced in 1989 to remind the public of potential risks:

> 'GOVERNMENT WARNING: (1) According to the Surgeon General, women should not drink alcoholic beverages during pregnancy because of the risk of birth defects. (2) Consumption of alcoholic beverages impairs your ability to drive a car or operate machinery, and may cause health problems'.

Greenfield has reviewed evidence related to the impact of the United States warning labels. He concluded that, after five years' exposure of the warning about drinking during pregnancy, almost half of US drinkers recalled the message. Comparable recall of the warning about drinking and driving was lower, at 26%. He concluded :

'the appropriate groups are being reminded of the harms, and that, other personal characteristics including drinking variables accounted for, those more exposed to the message appear more likely than others to be adopting harm-reduction strategies related to drinking and driving, and possibly drinking less per occasion when pregnant and having more conversations about drinking and pregnancy'. [22, p. 118]

During 1989, Tesco, a group of supermarkets in the United Kingdom, introduced the practice of providing information about the 'unit' content of alcoholic beverages. In 1999, a number of large producers of alcohol beverages in the United Kingdom announced that they were to begin to label bottles and cans with information about their alcohol content in 'units' of alcohol. Units have been widely used in the United Kingdom by researchers and in health-promotion campaigns. A United Kingdom unit, smaller than standard drinks in many other countries, contains 1 centilitre/7.9 g of alcohol. Each unit is equivalent to a bar measure of spirits, a glass of wine or half a pint of medium strength beer, lager, cider or stout. Stockwell and Single [55] have reviewed the use of 'standard unit labelling'. Such labelling may clearly be of value as an adjunct to informing people and promoting discussion about advisable and inadvisable levels of alcohol consumption. In the United Kingdom, for example, a number of bodies have for some years been providing advice about low-risk and high-risk drinking in relation to 'units' [56, 57]. As emphasized by Stockwell and Single, labelling is complicated by the confusing variety of strengths of alcoholic drinks and by international variation in what constitutes a 'standard drink'. They reported that Australian evidence suggests that the use of unit labels helps drinkers to assess more accurately the strength/alcohol-content of drinks. Stockwell and Single concluded as follows:

'There is a strong case for the introduction of unit labelling on both consumer and health grounds. With increasing medical knowledge regarding the adverse and beneficial effects of different patterns of alcohol use it is increasingly important that consumers are given the information they need to drink within limits of their choosing'. [55, p. 100]

Labelling can clearly increase factual awareness and, more important, appears to have increased the adoption of harm minimization by those most at risk, the heavier drinkers. Care must be taken to avoid inaccurate or misleading messages. In addition, countries vary greatly in the type of message that can be used and its political acceptability.

TREATMENT

Thom [58] has recently emphasized that the organization of clinical services for problem drinkers has changed over the past four decades. Some countries have a variety of treatment agencies, philosophies and approaches. Others, such as the USA, place great emphasis upon Alcoholics Anonymous/Minnesota Model/ Twelve-Step abstinence-oriented programmes, which view 'alcoholism' as an incurable disease. It is beyond the remit of this chapter to attempt to provide a detailed review or critique of the impact of the numerous therapeutic interventions for problem drinkers. A number of excellent studies already show convincingly that problem drinkers/alcoholics often improve dramatically after some form of intervention. Moreover, promising results have been achieved from different therapeutic approaches [59, 60]. Holder [61] has demonstrated that costs that individuals incur for health care are reduced after they receive therapeutic support for a drinking problem.

Edwards et al. [8, op cit.] have concluded that there is compelling evidence that a variety of personal interventions, sometimes brief and inexpensive, have helped to improve the lives of people with serious alcohol problems. Cameron [62] has stressed that services for people with severe drinking problems can be a valuable way of getting them through difficult periods of their lives. Such services are also likely to have a substantial impact on the well-being of family members, work associates and significant others.

Treatment for alcohol problems/alcohol dependence/alcoholism can be, and often is, 'effective'. In particular, it has been shown to help problem drinkers to stop or to reduce their heavy and harmful drinking. This has led to a reduction in adverse social consequences, such as harm to self, family, colleagues, friends and other social contacts. Countries vary greatly in the nature and range of their treatment and counselling services for problem drinkers. Even so, it appears that many, if not all, approaches often achieve very good results. Inexpensive, brief, interventions often appear to be highly productive, though some people may require extended support.

SUSTAINABILITY

A crucial factor in determining the value of any 'effective' harm minimization initiative is whether it can be sustained. Many activities that are in progress in the 'alcohol field' are not evaluated in any meaningful way. This is true of services provided to help and support 'problem drinkers' or 'alcoholics' or their families, as well as many community-based, regional or national initiatives. Sometimes there is even disagreement about what criteria are to be used to define 'effective impact'. In the United Kingdom, for example, it has been claimed that some past anti-drink–driving campaigns were successful because the number of positive breath tests had risen! Such rises may have indicated greater police vigilance or activity, but, regrettably, not a fall in intoxicated driving-behaviour. In fact, as reported by Stewart and Sweedler [63] and Plant and Cameron [4], alcohol-impaired driving has been declining in the United Kingdom as well as in many other countries. Even so, the reasons for the change in both attitudes and behaviour in relation to drinking and driving remain unclear. They have occurred under many different legal and policy jurisdictions. Graham et al. [64] have produced an invaluable guide to the assessment of client/clinical outcomes.

A number of past initiatives to reduce the level of alcohol-related problems have shown some clear signs of 'success', but have not been sustained. The short life of the Torquay venture, described by Jeffs and Saunders [34 op cit.], is an instance of this. It should be emphasized that some strategies may take a long time to become fully effective. Once a positive impact has been demonstrated, they should, to retain any value, be sustained. It seems that this often does not happen. This may be because of limited political commitment or the short attention spans of some policy-makers. Initiatives founder sometimes because key people, initiators or supporters, lose interest or move elsewhere. As Room et al. [65], have emphasized, social and political support are important factors in deciding whether a policy is retained.

Allamani et al. [30] have emphasized that some types of alcohol-related problem may take a long time to be reduced. Even gains achieved in a short time need to be maintained. Harm reduction, therefore, may require extended and sustained action. Ideally, successful strategies should be sustained by institutional means [66]. Moreover, effective initiatives are likely to require the implementation of a battery of separate but interrelated measures. An excellent instance of both effective and sustained community-wide action, from outside the alcohol field, as noted by Madden and Thornton [31], is the North Karelia Project in Finland, which reduced rates of heart disease by more than 70%. This was achieved by a comprehensive battery of community actions spanning a period of more than 20 years. It transformed both smoking and eating patterns in an area which, at the outset, had a catastrophic level of mortality from heart disease [67].

STRUCTURAL CONTROL POLICIES

This chapter is concerned mainly with harm minimization, as defined above. The potential of policies designed to regulate the extent of alcohol consumption and the availability of alcohol should also be acknowledged, however. As outlined by Godfrey [68] and Raistrick, Hodgson and Ritson [1, op cit.], alcohol taxation may be used to regulate alcohol consumption, but this is unlikely to be a popular approach; also, the relationship between price and consumption is less clear-cut than has sometimes been assumed. Nuisance may be reduced by policies that regulate the number and operation of licensed alcohol outlets.

Establishments with bad records in this regard should be closely monitored and, if necessary, closed. The Government of the United Kingdom has recently proposed this approach, for example.

CONCLUSION

Alcohol problems are not insurmountable. This does not mean that they will ever be totally eradicated. There are proven ways of reducing them, however, given the requisite political will or social pressure. Table 1 summarizes some of this evidence.

Table 1 The impact of some strategies

Education
- Raises awareness
- Increases factual knowledge
- Changes attitudes

Community action
- Creates coalitions of concerned people
- Reduces alcohol-related crime and disorder
- Reduces alcohol-related injuries
- Enhances local amenities/quality of life
- May improve services for problem drinkers and their families
- Can respond to issues of local concern and local priorities

Safer drinking places
- Reduce intoxication and aggression
- Reduce accidental and non-accidental injuries

Labelling to warn and inform
- Increases awareness
- Raises factual knowledge
- Helps drinkers assess their consumption more accurately
- Heavier drinkers appear to adopt harm-minimizing strategies

Treatment
- Often helps problem drinkers reduce both consumption and related adverse social consequences
- Helps people survive difficult periods of their lives

Structural control policies
- Reduce rates of problem drinking
- May be unpopular

This chapter provides merely a brief and highly selective introduction to what is now a massive literature on a wide variety of ways in which alcohol-related problems may be curbed.

The minimization of the adverse social consequences of heavy and inappropriate drinking is likely to remain controversial. This is understandable, for people vary greatly in their views about alcohol and the consequences of its use. It is suggested that the most fruitful way of hacking through the jungles of vested interest and disagreement that often obscure the facts about policy options is to refer to four key questions noted earlier in this chapter:

- Have they worked?
- Are they transferable to other contexts?
- Are they politically and socially acceptable?
- Can they be sustained?

Fatalism is unjustified. It is re-emphasized that alcohol problems can be minimized if there is a will to do so.

REFERENCES

1. Raistrick, D. et al., eds. (1999) *Tackling Alcohol Together: The Evidence Base for a UK Alcohol Policy*, Free Association Books, London.
2. Single, E. (1999) *Future Policy Directions*, Verbal presentation in plenary session in Addictions Forum/Alcohol and Health Research Centre National Conference on Drugs: Health and Social Issues, Edinburgh.
3. Musto, D.F. (1997) Alcohol control in historical perspective, in *Alcohol: Minimising the Harm: What Works?* (eds M.A. Plant et al.), Free Association Books, London, pp. 10–25.
4. Plant, M.A. and Cameron, D., eds. (in press) *The Alcohol Report*, Free Association Books, London.
5. Bruun, K. et al. (1975) *Alcohol Control Policies in Public Health Perspective*, Finnish Foundation for Alcohol Studies, Helsinki.
6. Ledermann, S. (1956) *Alcool, Alcoolism, Alcoolisation* [Alcohol, Alcoholism, Alcoholisation], Presses Universitaires de France, Paris [1 and 2].
7. Kreitman, N. (1986) Alcohol consumption and the preventive paradox. *British Journal of Addiction* **81**, 353–363.
8. Edwards, G. et al. (1994) *Alcohol Policy and the Public Good*, Oxford University Press, Oxford.
9. WHO. (1992) *European Alcohol Action Plan*, World Health Organization Regional Office for Europe, Copenhagen.
10. Rehm, J. (1999) Draining the ocean to prevent shark attacks? *Nordic Studies on Alcohol and Drugs* **16** (English Supplement), 46–54.
11. Schilts, R. (1987) *And the Band Played On*, Penguin, Harmondsworth.
12. Gray, M. (1998) *Drug Crazy: How We Got into this Mess and How We Can Get Out*, Random House, New York.

13. Plant, E.J. and Plant, M.A. (1999) Primary prevention for young children: a comment on the UK government's 10 year drug strategy. *International Journal of Drug Policy* **10**, 385–401.
14. O'Hare, P. (1992) Preface: a note on the concept of harm reduction, in *The Reduction of Drug-Related Harm* (eds P. O'Hare *et al.*), Tavistock/Routledge, London.
15. O'Hare, P. *et al.*, eds. (1992) *The Reduction of Drug-Related Harm*, Tavistock/Routledge, London.
16. Heather, N. *et al.*, eds. (1993) *Psychoactive Drugs and Harm Reduction: From Faith to Science*, Whurr Publishers, London.
17. Erickson, P.G. *et al.*, eds. (1997) *Harm Reduction: A New Direction for Drug Policies and Programs*, University of Toronto Press, Toronto.
18. Stockwell, T. et al. *Sharpening the Focus of Alcohol Policy from Aggregate Consumption to Harm and Risk Reduction*, Paper presented at the 22nd Alcohol Epidemiology Symposium, Kettil Bruun Society, Edinburgh, June 7th 1996.
19. Plant, M.A. *et al.*, eds. (1997) *Alcohol: Minimising the Harm: What Works?* Free Association Books, London.
20. Grant, M. and Litvak, J., eds. (1998) *Drinking Patterns and Their Consequences*, Taylor and Francis, Washington, DC.
21. Greenfield, T.K. and Kaskutas, L.A. (1994) *Changes in Public Opinion about Alcohol Control and Intervention Policies in the US: A Five Year Trend Study*, Paper presented at the American Public Health Association Annual Meeting, Washington, DC, October 30th–November 4th 1994.
22. Greenfield, T.K. (1997) Warning labels: evidence on harm reduction from long-term American surveys, in *Alcohol: Minimising the Harm: What Works?* (eds M.A. Plant *et al.*), Free Association Books, London, pp. 105–125.
23. Department of Health and Social Services. (1999) *Reducing Alcohol Related Harm in Northern Ireland*, DHSS Policy Development and Review Unit, Belfast.
24. Plant, M.A. and Plant, M.L. (1997) Alcohol education and harm minimisation, in *Alcohol: Minimising the Harm: What Works?* (eds M.A. Plant *et al.*), Free Association Books, London, pp. 193–210.
25. Clayton, R.R. *et al.* (1996) DARE (Drug Abuse Resistance Education): very popular but not very effective, in *Intervening With Drug-Involved Youth* (eds C.B. McCoy *et al.*), Sage Publications, London, pp. 101–109.
26. Dukes, R.L. *et al.* (1997) Long-term impact of drug abuse resistance education (DARE): result of a 6-year follow-up. *Evaluation Research* **21**, 483–500.
27. Lindström, P. and Svensson, R. (1998) Attitudes towards drugs among school youths: an evaluation of the Swedish DARE programme. *Nordic Studies on Alcohol and Drugs* **15**, 7–23.
28. Hawthorne, G. *et al.* (1996) Does life education's drug education programme have a public health benefit? *Addiction* **90**(2), 205–215.
29. Wright, L. (in press) Alcohol education, in *The Alcohol Report* (eds M.A. Plant and D. Cameron), Free Association Books, London.
30. Allamani, A. *et al.* (2000) Introduction: community action research and the prevention of alcohol problems at the local level. *Substance Use and Misuse* **35**, 1–10.
31. Madden, S. and Thornton, C. (1998) *Quality of Life and Sustainable Communities: What are Community Concerns?* Alcohol and Health Research Centre, Edinburgh, (Report for Forward Scotland).
32. Gilmour, C. (1999) *Personal communication*.
33. Paterson, F. (1994) *Evaluation of Public Drinking Bylaws in Scotland*, Paper presented at the 37th Scottish Alcohol Problems Research Symposium, Pitlochry, April 13th 1994.

34. Jeffs, B. and Saunders, W. (1983) Minimising alcohol-related offences by enforcement of existing legislation. *British Journal of Addiction* **78**, 67–78.
35. Ilgunas, M. (1994) *The Motherwell Experience*, Paper presented at the 37th Scottish Alcohol Problems Research Symposium, Pitlochry, April 13th 1994.
36. McKenzie, K. (1994) *The West Lothian Experience*, Paper presented at the 37th Scottish Alcohol Problems Research Symposium, Pitlochry, April 13th 1994.
37. Collins, J.J. (1982) *Drinking and Crime*, Tavistock, London
38. Saltz, R.F. (1997) Prevention where alcohol is sold and consumed, in *Alcohol: Minimising the Harm: What Works?* (eds M.A. Plant *et al.*), Free Association Books, London, pp. 72–84.
39. Homel, R. and Clark, J. (1994) The prediction and prevention of violence in pubs and clubs, in *Crime Prevention Studies* (ed. R.V. Clark), Criminal Justice Press, Monsey, New York.
40. Homel, R. *et al.* (1994) *The Impact of the Surfers Paradise Safety Action Project*, Centre for Crime Policy and Public Safety, School of Justice Administration, Griffith University. Nathan, Queensland.
41. Graham, K. and Homel, R. (1997) Creating safer bars, in *Alcohol: Minimising the Harm: What Works?* (eds M.A. Plant *et al.*), Free Association Books, London, pp. 171–192.
42. Holmila, M., ed. (1997) *Community Prevention of Alcohol Problems*, Macmillan, London.
43. Moskalewicz, J. and Swiatkiewicz, G. (2000) Malczyce, Poland: a multifaceted community action project in Eastern Europe in a time of rapid economic change. *Substance Use and Misuse* **35**(1 and 2), 189–202.
44. Graham, K. (1985) Determinants of heavy drinking and drinking problems: the contribution of the bar environment, in *Public Drinking and Public Policy* (eds E. Single and T. Storm), Addiction Research Foundation, Toronto.
45. Graham, K. *et al.* (1980) Aggression and bar room environments. *Journal of Studies on Alcohol* **4**, 277–292.
46. Graham, K. and Plant, M.A. (in press) Harm minimisation, in *The Alcohol Report* (eds M.A. Plant and D. Cameron), Free Association Books, London.
47. Cavan, S. *(1966) Liquor License: An Ethnography of Bar Behaviour*, Aldine, Chicago.
48. Single, E. and Storm, T., eds. (1984) *Public Drinking and Public Policy*, Addiction Research Foundation, Toronto.
49. Bach, P.J. and Schaefer, J.M. (1979) The tempo of country music and the rate of drinking in bars. *Journal of Studies on Alcohol* **40**, 1058–1059.
50. Kaufman, D. and Mahoney, J.M. (1999) The effects of waitresses' touch on alcohol consumption in dyads. *Journal of Social Psychology* **139**, 261–267.
51. Shepherd, J.P. *et al.* (1990) Glass abuse and urban licensed premises. *Journal of the Royal Society of Medicine* **83**, 276–277.
52. Shepherd, J.P. *et al.* (1991) Impact resistance of drinking glasses. *British Medical Journal* **303**, 133.
53. Plant, M.A. *et al.* (1994) No such thing as a safe glass. *British Medical Journal* **308**, 1237–1238.
54. Plant, M.A. and Mills, D. (1997) *Glass Conscious: Safer Glasses – Fewer Injuries?* Scientist, vol Spring, 1. The Faculty of Science and Engineering News, the University of Edinburgh, Edinburgh, 1994/5.
55. Stockwell, T. and Single, E. (1997) Standard unit labelling of alcohol containers, in *Alcohol: Minimising the Harm: What Works?* (eds M.A. Plant *et al.*), Free Association Books, London, pp. 85–104.
56. Royal College of Psychiatrists. (1979) *Alcohol and Alcoholism*, Tavistock, London.
57. Royal College of Psychiatrists. (1986) *Alcohol: Our Favourite Drug*, Tavistock, London.

58. Thom, B. (1999) *Dealing With Drink*, Free Association Books, London.
59. Project Match Research Group. (1997) Matching alcoholism treatments to client heterogeneity: Project Match post-treatments outcomes. *Journal of Studies on Alcohol* **58**, 7–29.
60. Heather, N. (in press) Psychosocial treatment approaches and the findings of Project Match, in *The Alcohol Report* (eds M.A. Plant and D. Cameron), Free Association Books, London.
61. Holder, H.D. (1987) Alcoholism treatment and patient health care cost saving. *Medical Care* **25**, 547–554.
62. Cameron, D. (1997) Keeping the customer satisfied: harm minimisation and clinical practice, in *Alcohol: Minimising the Harm: What Works?* (eds M.A. Plant *et al.*), Free Association Books, London, pp. 233–247.
63. Stewart, K. and Sweedler, B.M. (1997) Driving under the influence of alcohol, in *Alcohol: Minimising the Harm: What Works?* (eds M.A. Plant *et al.*), Free Association Books, London, pp. 126–142.
64. Graham, K. *et al.* (1995) *Directory of Client Outcome Measures, for Addiction Treatment Programmes*, Addiction Research Foundation, Toronto.
65. Room, R. *et al.* (1995) Trends in public opinion about alcohol policy initiatives in Ontario and the US: 1989–1991. *Drug and Alcohol Review* **14**, 35–47.
66. Holder, H.D. and Moore, R.S. (2000) Institutionalisation of community action projects to reduce alcohol-use related problems: systematic facilitators. *Substance Use and Misuse* **35**, 75–86.
67. Puska, P. *et al.*, eds. (1995) *The North Karelia Project: 20 Years Results and Experiences*, National Public Health Institute, Helsinki.
68. Godfrey, C. (1997) Can tax be used to minimise harm? A health economist's perspective, in *Alcohol: Minimising the Harm: What Works?* (eds M.A. Plant *et al.*), Free Association Books, London, pp. 29–42.

Chapter eleven

Community initiatives as strategies for implementation of the European Alcohol Action Plan

M. Holmila

INTRODUCTION

The European Alcohol Action Plan recognizes the importance of community programmes and local action in promoting healthy lifestyles as well as in securing public and political support for modifying the sale and consumption of alcohol. In addition to developing local policy, local action can exert a powerful influence on national and even international policy. The Action Plan recommends that greater effort be put into encouraging, strengthening and supporting local action [1, p. 14].

In modern times, many countries have adopted national policies in response to public concern about alcohol abuse. Locally initiated action became especially important in the late 20th century as countries or regions entered into free trade agreements and international action removed barriers to the flow of goods between countries. The result has been erosion of well-established national policies that had been designed to reduce alcohol-related health and social problems. Local initiatives have thus become even more critical. Local policies also provide some protection against the full impact of a substantial weakening of national policies. In the Scandinavian countries, for example, national-level policy on preventing alcohol abuse and controlling alcohol

---

Harald Klingemann and Gerhard Gmel (eds.), Mapping the Social Consequences of Alcohol Consumption, 161–170.
© *2001 Kluwer Academic Publishers. Printed in Great Britain.*

consumption has been weakened and there is a growing need for municipal action.

External factors, therefore, have led to the strengthening of the role of community action in harm reduction in relation to alcohol, but community action by its nature is very well suited to this role. As Holder and Giesbrecht [2] have pointed out, it is logical to use an approach that draws on community organization and social reform to counter and prevent alcohol-related harm, since such harm is a consequence of social behaviour often associated with institutional contexts and has strong cultural restraints and inducements.

Community action can also constitute an alternative to a modernist, rational approach in which a state-level intervention is believed to act uniformly to reduce harm and is seen as sufficient. Community action being non-linear can be responsive to the diverse needs of different community sectors and to changing circumstances [3, p. 61].

Harmful consequences of alcohol use affect the local community directly. They include street and home violence related to intoxication, disorder in public places, damage to property, litter, noise made by drunken people, and the daily exposure of children to heavy drinking in their neighbourhoods. Police, teachers, doctors and social workers in most communities report on the damaging long-lasting effects of drinking on the well-being of children, families and entire communities.

What is community-based prevention?

Community-based prevention may be defined as an attempt to coordinate the resources of a community to prevent alcohol-related harm. As such, it is not new. In relation to alcohol and drug use it has a long history. It is only over the last ten years or so, however, that experts have reported on, evaluated or discussed the subject, and only relatively recently that it has become a topic of international scientific discussion. Much has been learned during this short period, however, and the potential of community action and its links with state and international action are now better recognized. Past projects have built up a rich store of experience in developing and sustaining local initiatives to reduce problems. Some of the lessons learned in international discussion on community-based prevention can now be summarized. Research on community-based initiatives has done much to clarify, evaluate and disseminate these experiences.

Scientists have pointed out that the community approach to prevention requires a paradigm shift. Such a shift demands more than simply adding the word 'community' to the prevention vocabulary. Effective strategies of community-level alcohol policies will often be quite different from those of national policies, and their development will require a different point of view or perspective. According to Holder [4, p. 13], neither the individualistic nor the deterministic prevention perspective in community-based work will achieve results. The individualistic approach disregards the environment and cultural and social circumstances. It is concerned with individuals at risk rather than with the community; yet the community needs to be the focus of the prevention. The deterministic approach produces a defined outcome, without regard to the complexities of community life or community systems. Community-based interventions, however, alter the social, cultural, economic and physical environment in ways that modify or counter in varied and not always predictable ways the conditions that favour the occurrence of alcohol-related problems.

Problems arise basically from a community's way of life or its circumstances, not from the characteristics of some of its individual members. Individuals have their own impact, but curing or removing a problem individual will not result in sustainable reduction in harm related to the use of alcohol and drugs if the community dynamics that gave rise to these problems are not influenced. Unless environmental changes are made, new individuals will always replace those who are seen as problem individuals. Policies developed in the local environment have a longer-lasting effect than individually oriented educational or treatment programmes, and thus are usually more economical.

Many of the forces that give rise to problems in the community cannot be influenced at the community level, however. Wider economic trends and international trade agreements, for instance, can affect the well-being of a local community, or the availability of alcohol in the community. Community-level action can do little to counter such influences. It is crucial to be able to distinguish factors that can be influenced by community action from those that cannot.

Communities are complex systems, which adjust to interventions. Any environmental intervention can have unexpected or negative effects in relation to the prevention of problems arising from the use of alcohol or drugs. It is essential to the effectiveness of local action groups, and critical to international scientific evaluation of community-based prevention, that such processes are analysed and understood.

Action should be based on issues of local concern

The success of local action is dependent upon a cooperative process of problem recognition and it may need to be repeated frequently in the course of a project. Information on local policy arrangements, drinking practices, and key aspects of local drinking cultures and drinking-related problems should be obtained, as far as possible, from a variety of sources, such as surveys, interviews with community representatives, archival data and official statistics.

Local participants decide on priorities among the goals and means of action. They need access, however, to research-based knowledge of how problems are related to one another, and what previous community programmes or other communities have been able to achieve.

The community organization model provides a structured, five-phase guide or process (analysis, design, implementation, maintenance and evaluation) for achieving community action goals. In practice, community organization is often seen as the key strategy whereby citizens, organizations and communities are mobilized for health action and promoting conditions for change. Essentially, this mobilization should give them a sense of ownership of the programme and, as an outcome, increased problem-solving abilities and competence in dealing with threats to health and well-being [5].

Diversity in the European experience

Different societies implement community-based programmes within different organizational settings and cultural and ideological contexts. In Scandinavia, municipalities are encouraged to develop their own preventive programmes [6, 7]. Many Eastern European countries are experiencing systemic transformation and radical changes in their political, social and moral orders as well as at the local level [8, p. 1]. Much community-based prevention is never reported; its occurrence as a part of a research project is exceptional in this respect.

EXAMPLES OF REPORTED EUROPEAN PROJECTS

The Lahti project

The Lahti Project, on the prevention of alcohol-related harm, was conducted in Lahti, Finland, from the autumn of 1992 until 1995 [9, 10]. It covered most sectors of the community and was coordinated through the city's health bureau. The work was organized into modules corresponding to the following activities: identifying alcohol problems in the community, group interviews of key persons, education and information, secondary prevention in health care, social support for heavy drinkers and family members, influencing the supply of alcohol, and evaluation. The core of the project consisted of seven researchers, information experts, and the local coordinator. Programme evaluation showed some community-level effects: the project succeeded in raising among the public an awareness of alcohol problems and knowledge of facts about alcohol and alcohol-related harm; it received extensive media coverage, and it reached its target groups, in particular the heavy drinkers. Also, it created new, permanent forms of social response to alcohol problems, and helped to create new networks and forms of cooperation between various public sectors and voluntary organizations.

The Florence Community Alcohol Action Research project

This project began in 1992 with the aim of creating community awareness of the risks associated with the drinking of wine and other alcoholic drinks [11]. It was divided into four interacting components: a public-information component, which promoted a healthy lifestyle and proposed the idea of 'responsible drinking'; a community school programme aimed at increasing awareness of health issues in relation to alcoholic beverages and food; training of primary-health-care professionals in early detection of high-risk drinkers; and training in alcohol-problem issues of volunteers who helped in the transport of injured people to hospital emergency rooms. The municipal administration appointed a coordinating committee for healthy lifestyles, which included 17 local institutions and associations, to promote further community-led initiatives for the prevention of alcohol-related problems.

The Kirseberg project

The Kirseberg Project, carried out in Malmö, Sweden between 1988 and 1996 [12], integrated many aspects of community-based models for prevention of heart disease. The project employed a community-wide strategy, built on a combination of methods, designed to achieve small but sustained changes in the drinking habits of the majority of the population; it included small-scale programmes directed at schools, health-care organizations and other sub-populations to attain more intensive and profound changes in drinking. During its final year it introduced measures to decrease access to alcohol. When the project ended in 1996 the Kirseberg city council took over responsibility for its organization and its preventive activities. The project reached around two-thirds of the population of Kirseberg and alcohol was identified as the main issue in relation to heart disease.

The Malczyce Community Action project in Poland

The Malczyce project was a one-year demonstration project on prevention of drug misuse, carried out in a local community during an economic crisis in 1994–1995 [13]. Its major outcome was a Prevention and Community Action Package, which summarized the experiences accumulated during its implementation. Locally, the project sought to ensure sustainability by forming a local prevention lobby.

The Stad project in Stockholm, Sweden

This is an action-oriented project with a ten-year perspective, funded by the county and city councils. Three areas for prevention were chosen: secondary prevention in health care, youth programmes, and server training in restaurants. The long-term goal is to achieve policy changes in policies and structures [14].

Those examples are from Europe. More examples could be given from other parts of the world, in particular from the United States, Canada and New Zealand. The five projects presented above range in duration from one year to as long as ten years; some target alcohol, some illegal drugs and some both, but all five use a multi-method approach and aim at activating the entire community and bringing about structural and environmental changes.

LESSONS LEARNED

Wide participation

Common to all community programmes is wide inter-sectorial networking and co-operation. Most local action programmes have therefore involved key community players – the police, licensing inspectors, restaurant owners, schools, youth workers, voluntary associations and the health and social sector. Naturally, different societies, even different localities, vary as to who accept the important responsibilities in local undertakings. Most local action groups that have been described in the scientific literature have included professionals as their key members. Grass-roots movements, which are based only on citizen initiatives, have not been reported so often. It is to be expected that many citizens' movements, which can be of short duration or hardly visible, simply fail to attract the attention of researchers or the public.

As local action is typically based on networks of people with very different backgrounds, the networks are faced with the task of finding a common language and common goals. The project co-ordinator's role is crucial in this sometimes complicated process. It must be recognized that community activists will have to deal with many conflicting interests as well as with institutions and sectors that are potential partners in community action.

Even if cultural, political and local circumstances vary as to what kind of local action is feasible and effective, international networking and exchange of experiences has proven to be most important for developing the field. During the past decade a network of scientists and practitioners interested in community-based prevention research has been created globally and within Europe.

The European network has arranged two large conferences with the support of the European Commission and the World Health Organization Regional Office for Europe. The First European Symposium on Community Action Programmes to Prevent Alcohol Problems took place at Malmö, Sweden [15]. The Second European Symposium was held in Portugal in 1999. Also, the WHO Regional Office for Europe, through its Healthy Cities network, has promoted community-based prevention of problems related to alcohol and drug use.

Before these conferences, four international meetings were held on research on local programmes for preventing harm related to alcohol, the first at Scarborough, Ontario, Canada in 1989 [16]; the second in San Diego, California in 1992 [17]; the third at Greve in Chianti, Italy, in September 1995 [18]; and the fourth in New Zealand, in 1998 [19]. From these meetings, networks have been established or strengthened and publications have been issued giving shape and content to local work, which so often is difficult to comprehend under the conditions of everyday work.

Sustainability is a challenge

Despite the enthusiasm, energy and good intentions of those who work in and support prevention, unless prevention becomes a part of the routine and regular processes of the community the long-term value of their efforts is often lost [20]. Thus, even if the programmes that initiated prevention activities in a community are not themselves sustained, they should be used to introduce and institutionalize policy and structural measures that improve the community's health and well-being [21, p. 75].

The basic requirement for the institutionalization of community prevention is that the community must accept and sustain the activities that are designed to reduce problems. This is not always easy; preventive measures can disrupt a community's social and economic arrangements. Local action may, for instance, want to impose restrictions on alcohol outlets associated with disorder and violence in the neighbourhood, but some inhabitants and retailers are likely to oppose such measures as restrictions of their freedom. A local action group may want an increase in the resources allocated to preventive work, but the treatment providers may argue for more funds for expanding treatment services. As a result of social disorder caused by addicts drinking in the streets and parks, community representatives may suggest the provision of a shelter or a special day-time home for them, but local residents may object to it being sited in their vicinity, and a suitable location may be difficult to find.

There is so far little research-based knowledge about what keeps community action projects alive after original funding has ended and the researchers have left. Information about the stability of changes achieved and how best to maintain them is limited [22, pp. 1009–111]. Also, institutionalization or sustainability has rarely been an explicit primary objective of community action projects carried out up to now [4, p. 83].

One factor worth mentioning for its contribution to the institutionalization of community action projects is the cumulative effect of multiple prevention programmes operating on a variety of levels from the local to the international. Also, expert networks and scientific work have an important role to play in helping to build the experience and making it a sustainable part of national plans and structures, for instance.

The role of research in accumulating knowledge and experience

Scientific evaluation of community-level projects is an important part of developing the field. It is necessary to accumulate research-based information on the kinds of action that are likely to produce results. Community-based prevention provides an interesting challenge for evaluation methodology.

Quasi-experimental methods are not applicable in the conditions in which community programmes operate. Quasi-experimental evaluation requires full control of an intervention, its delivery and the context in which it is implemented. By definition, however, community programmes operate in complex and changing contexts. The hypothesis that community programmes are effective cannot, therefore, be ruled out despite the lack of sufficient supporting evidence [12, p. 81].

Positive results from quasi-experimental evaluation of community programmes (comparing experimental and control areas) have generally been within the range of random variations resulting from secular trends [23]. In only a few community-based prevention projects has outcome evaluation shown reduction in community aggregate indicators of alcohol problems [10, 24]. It may be that community programmes cannot add significantly to secular trends. Conventional statistical methods, however, may not easily detect small effects, though small effects can have important public health implications [25]. Also, local efforts that seek to reduce acute problems are likely to produce effects sooner than interventions directed at life-style problems such as hazardous levels of consumption. Besides showing outcome results, evaluation should contribute to understanding the processes that led or failed to lead to results, and the contexts and circumstances that affected the nature of those processes. This usually requires various types of data-gathering methods, including qualitative methods, as well as theoretical generalizations of the character of community processes. On the whole, evaluation of community-based processes is a challenging and interesting area within a social science that aims at understanding the nature of human communities.

Researchers, above all, are expected to produce a generalizable body of knowledge on the potential of community action. At the same time, within the research process, their interaction with practitioners in community projects, and the constant exchange of different kinds of knowledge, can contribute significantly to the development of community action.

The ten years of scientific discussion on community-based prevention of alcohol-related harm has revealed many instances of its usefulness and feasibility. The emphasis recently has been largely on the search for methods of achieving sustainability as well as for more detailed information on the effectiveness of different types of working instruments available to communities.

REFERENCES

1. WHO (1992). *European Alcohol Action Plan*, World Health Organization Regional Office for Europe, Copenhagen.
2. Holder, H.D. and Giesbrecht, N. (1990) Perspectives on the community action research, in *Research, Action and the Community: Experiences in the Prevention of Alcohol and Other Drug Problems* (eds N. Giesbrecht *et al.*), US Department of Health and Human Services, Rockville, MD, pp. 27–40 (OSAP Prevention Monograph 4).
3. Casswell, S. (2000) A decade of community action research. *Substance Use and Misuse* 35(1 and 2), 55–74.
4. Holder, H.D. (1998) *Alcohol and the Community. A Systems Approach to Prevention. International Research Monograph on Addictions*, Cambridge University Press, Cambridge.
5. Bracht, N., ed. (1990) *Health Promotion at the Community Level*, Sage Publications, Newbury Park, CA.
6. National Institute of Public Health 70 (1995) *National Plan of Action for Prevention of Alcohol Related Harm and Drug Abuse in Sweden*, Wassbergs Tryckeri, Stockholm.
7. The Finnish Ministry of Social Affairs and Health (1997) *Onks tietoo? Esitys kansallisen alkoholiohjelman toimeenpanemiseksi* [Suggestions for the implementation of the National Alcohol Action Plan]. Raittius- ja päihdeasiain neuvottelukunta. Sosiaali- ja terveysministeriön monisteita 14. Sosiaaali-ja terveysministeriö, The Finnish Ministry of Social Affairs and Health.
8. Sierolawski, J. *Drug and Alcohol Policy in Poland. Between Myths and Scientific Knowledge*, Paper presented at the Nordic Council on Alcohol and Drugs Meeting 'Knowledge and Expertise in Alcohol and Drug Policy', Bergen, 23–25 September 1999.
9. Holmila, M. (1995) Community action on alcohol: experiences of the Lahti project in Finland. *Health Promotion International* 10(4), 283–291.
10. Holmila, M., ed. (1997) *Community Prevention of Alcohol Problems*, Macmillan, London.
11. Allamani, A. *et al.* (2000) Alcohol carousel and children's school drawings as part of a community educational strategy. *Substance Use and Misuse* 35(1 and 2), 126–127.
12. Hanson, B.S. *et al.* (2000) Time trends in alcohol habits. Results from the Kirseberg Project in Malmö, Sweden. *Substance Use and Misuse* 35(1 and 2), 171–187.
13. Moskalewicz, J. and Swiatkiewicz, G. (2000) Malczyce, Poland: a multifaceted community action project in Eastern Europe in a time of rapid economic change. *Substance Use and Misuse* 35(1 and 2), 189–202.
14. Andréasson, S. *et al.* (1999) Exploring new roads to prevention of alcohol and other drug problems in Sweden: the STAD project, in *Kettil Bruun Society Thematic Meeting, Fourth Symposium on Community Action Research and the Prevention of Alcohol and Other Drug Problems* (eds S. Casswell *et al.*), Auckland, University of Auckland, Alcohol and Public Health Research Unit, Auckland.
15. Larsson, S. and Hanson, B.S., eds. (1999) *Community Based Alcohol Prevention in Europe – Research and Evaluation*, Proceedings of the First European Symposium on Community Action Programmes to Prevent Alcohol, European Commission, Studentlitteratur, Lund.
16. Giesbrecht, N. *et al.* (1990) *Research, Action and the Community: Experiences in the Prevention of Alcohol and Other Drug Problems*, Department of Health and Human Services, Office for Substance Abuse Prevention, Rockville, MD.
17. Greenfield, T.K. and Zimmermann, R., eds. (1993) *Experiences with Community Action Projects: New Research in the Prevention of Alcohol and Other Drug Problems.*

US Department of Health and Human Services, Rockville, MD, (CSAP Prevention Monograph 14).
18. Kettil Bruun Society (1995) *Community Action to Prevent Alcohol Problems*, Paper presented at the Third Symposium on Community Action Research, Greve in Chianti, Italy, 25–29 September 1995.
19. Casswell, S. et al., eds. (1999) *Kettil Bruun Society Thematic Meeting, Fourth Symposium on Community Action Research and the Prevention of Alcohol and other Drug Problems*, University of Auckland, Alcohol and Public Health Research Unit, Auckland.
20. Renauld, L. et al. (1997) L'institutionnalisation des programmes communautaires: revue de modèles théoriques et proposition d'un modèle. *Canadian Journal of Public Health* [Institutionalization of community programs: review of theoretical models and proposal of a model] **88**(2), 109–133.
21. Holder, H.D. and Moore, R.S. (2000) Institutionalisation of community action projects to reduce alcohol-use related problems: systematic facilitators. *Substance Use and Misuse* **35**, 75–86.
22. Bush, R. (1997) Can we achieve sustainable reduction in harms in local communities? *Drug and Alcohol Review* **16**, 1009–1011.
23. Winkleby, M. (1994) The future of community-based cardiovascular disease intervention studies. *American Journal of Public Health* **84**, 1369–1372.
24. Holder, H.D. (1997) A community prevention trial to reduce alcohol-involved trauma. *Addiction* **92**(2),155–171.
25. Fishbein, M. (1996) Great expectations or do we ask too much from community level interventions? *American Journal of Public Health* **86**, 1075–1076.